Sustainable Beauty

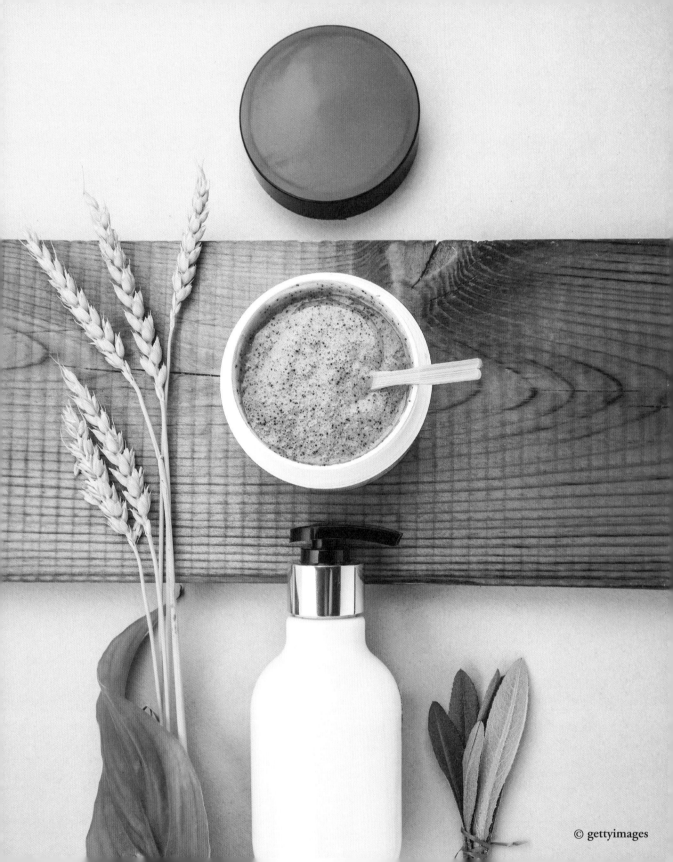

Sustainable Beauty

DIY Bath & Body Products for *Glowing Skin* & a *Greener Earth*

Ruchita Acharya

creative mind behind *Glow & Green*

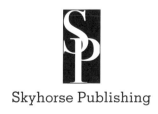

Skyhorse Publishing

Skyhorse Publishing books may be purchased in bulk at special discounts for sales promotion, corporate gifts, fund-raising, or educational purposes. Special editions can also be created to specifications. For details, contact the Special Sales Department, Skyhorse Publishing, 307 West 36th Street, 11th Floor, New York, NY 10018 or info@skyhorsepublishing.com.

Skyhorse® and Skyhorse Publishing® are registered trademarks of Skyhorse Publishing, Inc.®, a Delaware corporation.

Visit our website at www.skyhorsepublishing.com.

10 9 8 7 6 5 4 3 2 1

Library of Congress Cataloging-in-Publication Data is available on file.

Cover design by David Ter-Avanesyan
Cover photos by Dillip Jetti Photography

Print ISBN: 978-1-5107-7551-0
Ebook ISBN: 978-1-5107-7553-4

Printed in China

Special thanks to Kunal and Neev

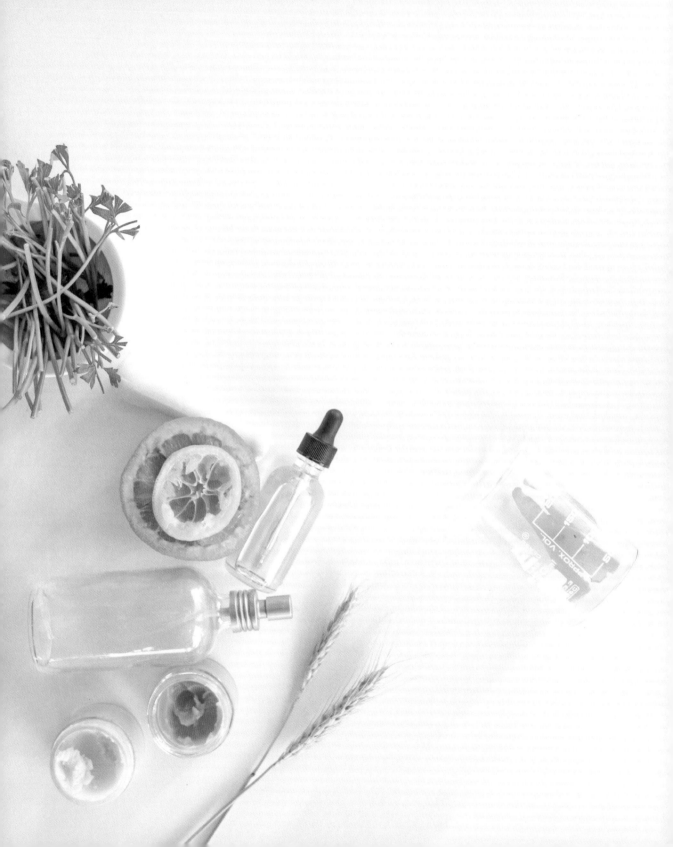

CONTENTS

PART 1

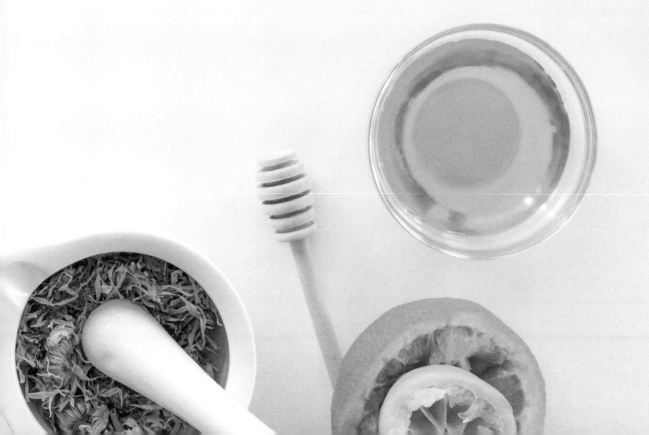

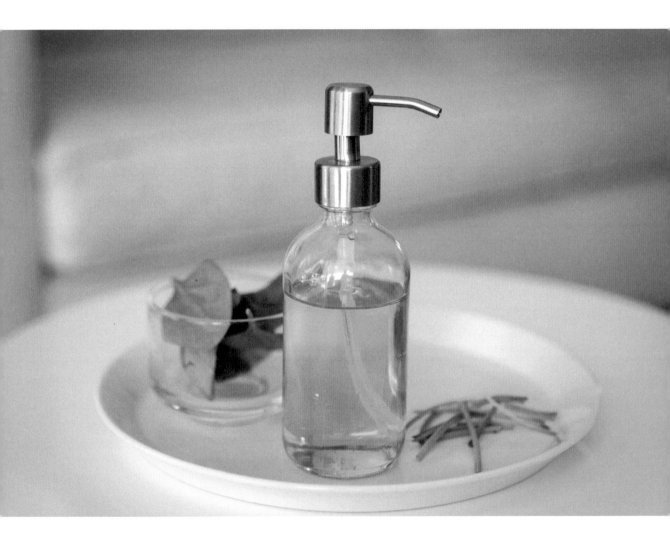

Chapter 1

DIY Sustainable Beauty in the Kitchen Using Food Scraps

At the most basic level of sustainable and clean living, it's common knowledge that buying and consuming locally sourced food is good for us. We know that we should check and double-check all the ingredients on our food labels. It's become second nature to buy organic vegetables and fruit from farmers' markets, put them into our juicer, and sip our smoothies from biodegradable or reusable jars. By participating in these activities, we proudly claim we are abiding by farm-to-table concepts. But in the flurry of mashing organic bananas for batches of Sunday morning keto pancakes, we as consumers often overlook the connection between sustainability and beauty.

That's why we're here: to learn about the missing piece to your sustainable lifestyle: a farm-to-beauty cabinet. When we buy or dine farm-to-table, we think we are saving our planet from greenhouse gas emissions and promoting the organic food chain while also getting healthy. But we can't ignore all the ways, as humans, that we *consume*. It's not just food that we take in from the environment. To lead a sustainable lifestyle, we must extend it to all aspects of our lives. We must have a transparent and sustainable beauty chain as well.

What Sustainable Really Means

Sustainable beauty means *understanding* beauty products—and not just in terms of good versus harmful ingredients. We should think of sustainable beauty in the same way that we think about our food, using a holistic approach (i.e., understanding how far commercial ingredients travel from production to shelf to hand, the pollution produced in our environment, and so on).

We are all aware that our planet is deteriorating. However, sustainable beauty is not just about using ethical manufacturing processes, fair-trade ingredients, and recycled packaging. It's also about understanding the true meaning of the American proverb, *We do not inherit the earth from our ancestors. Instead, we borrow it from our children.* If we keep this in mind and follow the principles outlined in this book, we can solve and resolve major environmental problems such as food waste, water accessibility, and more—all while doing good for ourselves by using good products.

Contrary to outdated beliefs, sustainable beauty products are effective. They comprise simple, natural, clean, and environmentally beneficial ingredients. Just as we consume fresh local fruits and vegetables to make our bodies healthier, sustainable beauty uses our beauty routine to nourish our skin and hair using fresh, local ingredients. The sustainable beauty product provides a perfect balance of safety to people and the planet and, in my opinion, should be economically viable for the consumer.

My Own Discovery

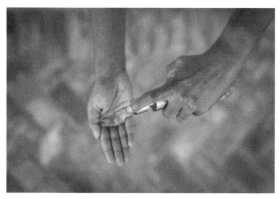

I grew up in a middle-class working family in India with a mom who never let me buy conventional beauty products. Instead, she taught me all the tips, tricks, and do-it-yourself (DIY) concoctions she used to avoid visiting salons and beauty stores. "Ruchita," she'd say,

"why bother sitting for hours in a salon when we have everything we need here for free?" Her reason was not *just* to save money. She legitimately believed that instead of lathering unknown chemicals on our skin, we should use the clean, green, ancient, and effective ingredients we already had. Thanks to natural food scraps, these ingredients were easily accessible in our kitchen pantry. Sustainability was not a well-known term in the nineties, but now, as I'm in my thirties, I can see that she taught me all those sustainability life lessons I didn't even realize I was getting.

Moving from a small Indian town to New York City at age twenty-three, I was cautiously hopeful that my life would improve because of my new opportunities for study. Suddenly, without my mom for the first time in my life, I became responsible for all the choices in my life—and my beauty and wellness routines were no exception. *Which beauty products should I buy? What's inside those beauty products? How many times should I go to the salon?* This may seem normal to Americans, but this newfound freedom presented a tricky situation in my life.

Flying high on convenience and variety, I bought many conventional beauty products and applied them to my skin without much consideration. I suddenly ignored individual ingredients and clung to generalizations, such as "If it's free from sulfate, it's good for me. If it's free from parabens, it's good for me."

Even though I felt conscious about clean beauty—avoiding parabens, sulfates, and the like—I still experienced skin and hair issues: acne, dehydrated skin, hair loss, greying hair, and brittle nails. Eventually, my efforts weren't enough. It often felt that the products I bought to fix my skin weren't doing anything they promised on the packaging.

Working in New York City as a sustainable program manager, I managed various projects based on green, clean, and sustainable principles after graduating from the New Jersey Institute of Technology. Even though I faced minor skin and hair issues during those years, I never connected my personal care and beauty products to my challenges. At age thirty-two, I moved to the west coast, and those minor skin and hair issues became amplified.

Shortly afterward, I suffered a miscarriage, a painful yet eye-opening incident in my life. An overwhelming and emotional time for me, I decided it was time to brave up and look closely at choices affecting my overall wellness, including what was in my cabinet full of beauty products. When I looked closely, I was disappointed and sad. What were these long lists with ingredients I didn't even recognize? Were these products performing the way they had been marketed? How had I disconnected from my mother's teaching?

After losing the baby, I was at a breaking point in my life. Professionally, I shifted into working in landfill and solid waste management. Since landfills are not isolated, they are connected to the environment—so whatever gets dumped affects the whole environment around it. I saw firsthand how many plastic-based unused beauty products ended up in landfills and in our waterways. I came to know the dark side of beauty.

Beauty Pollution

Not until then did I know that microbeads and microplastics (like glitters) are not soluble in water, thus polluting the ocean and its marine life. I didn't know that avobenzone, an ingredient common in sunscreen, is harmful to coral reefs. I learned that artificial fragrances, hair mist, and hairspray pollute the air. In addition, many beauty products consist of palm oil, which has led to significant deforestation. According to a study by Zero Waste Europe, our use of beauty and personal care products produced 142 billion packaging units in 2018 alone. This only added to the total energy utilized and the giant carbon footprint caused by transporting ingredients and finished goods.

As a sustainability professional and beauty addict myself, I had to conclude that what I was slathering all over my face and body (and paying a crazy amount of money for) was not only harmful to myself and my surroundings but likely ineffective. It was enough to shake me into action.

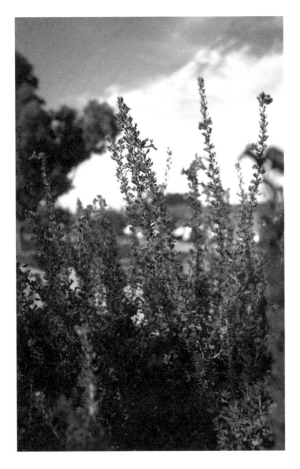

1. Use only clean formulas
2. Understand the supply chain of each ingredient, called "beauty miles traveled"
3. Abide by the motto *Must be good for the skin and good for the environment*

It didn't take long before I faced a decision. I could go on researching and checking every single ingredient in commercial products to understand the supply chain of those ingredients and their impact on my body, or I could try to replicate this process in the kitchen as my mom taught me to do in the first place—using simple pantry items and food scraps.

During my childhood, my mom and grandmother used to dry mango seeds and make powder from them for their beauty rituals. Adding this powder to your face masks brightens your skin tone. They also taught me that the leftover water from making rice or lentils could be used as an effective hair rinse or facial toner. It's good for you and the environment, as you upcycle food scraps.

That's how I began. And that's how we'll begin together, too. We have everything we need to make sustainable beauty products in our kitchens.

Let's Talk about Your Journey

I'm here to show you how making your personal care products is not only doable but also

My Solution

From my home in the Bay Area, I studied at Formula Botanica, a London-based beauty school. Whatever I learned, I decided I would share with conscious consumers like me, who were realizing the importance of green and sustainable beauty. With this intention, my company, *Glow & Green*, was born. I committed to buying only products aligned with these three principles:

an enjoyable and therapeutic process. What you'll be learning in this book is the equivalent of healthy meal prep—but for your face and skin—for the whole week. As a result, you'll save money and, more importantly, have complete control over your beauty regimen.

This book is a result of my endless hours of study, sustainability knowledge, practice, and a diploma in organic skin-care formulation.

But even more, it's the shortcut to all my tried-and-true beauty recipes. By the end of our journey, you will understand how to create your own sustainable and eco-conscious lifestyle. With my recipes, you will not just solve your own beauty problems, but will also solve significant sustainability issues such as food waste and water accessibility, too.

Let's get glowing and go green.

Chapter 2

Better the Shelf: Designing Effective DIY Recipes for Beauty and Well-Being

DIY beauty is often considered less potent or less powerful than commercial products. Many people believe that if a product is manufactured by a factory and sold at beauty stores at expensive rates, the product will be effective. This leads them to spend a lot of money on store-bought products which may not work better than what they create at home.

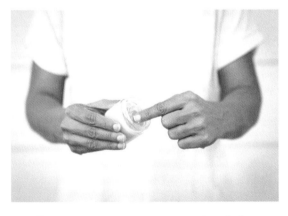

On average, most conventional beauty products are made up of 30+ ingredients. These ingredients often come from a supply chain containing carbon emissions. Not only is this not sustainable for our planet, but it is certainly not sustainable for our bodies. With DIY beauty, I always know what's inside my jar.

Popular beauty brands spend most of their budget on marketing instead of on making the product itself. I still remember when I met one beauty executive from one of the renowned brands at a party, and she happily confessed that 60–70 percent of their product cost is associated with packaging and marketing. The ingredients are dirt cheap, and anyone can create them in their own kitchen.

If we methodically implement DIY beauty, we can create luxurious skin- and body-care products. In this chapter, I want to share pointers and tips to help you create better skin-care formulas than what's on the market. I truly believe that if we know how to make an effective homemade product, we will feel so luxurious and empowered by what we can make by ourselves in the comfort of our homes that we will stop wasting our money on manufactured beauty products.

Before we go any further, let me share my own experience. As a beauty enthusiast myself, when I started my DIY beauty journey, I became overexcited, rushed to my kitchen, and mixed a bunch of products together. Due to my excitement, I measured nothing, so when I tried to make the same recipe again, I was lost.

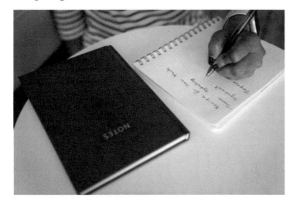

I don't want you to make the same mistake I did, so before making these recipes, you first need to understand the basic categories of beauty products: foundational ingredients, functional ingredients, active ingredients, aromatic ingredients, and aesthetic ingredients. These ingredients work hand in hand to give you the best skin treatment you can ask for without negative side effects. My ultimate goal for you is to make DIY sustainable skin-care products that are just as effective (if not more!) than conventional beauty products.

Let's Talk about Designing DIY Skin Care

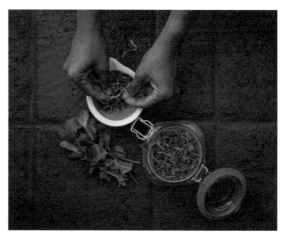

In making the beauty recipes for this book, I adopted the same method I learned while studying skin-care formulation and have outlined the steps you should follow when embarking on your own DIY beauty journey! If you follow this three-step process and put your recipes to pen and paper, you will have access to better products than your favorite beauty brand.

1. Figure out the base of the product
You have two choices for your base: An oil base such as butter, wax, or oils, or a water base such as glycerin, hydrosols, tinctures, etc. There shouldn't be any rush to go to your kitchen; instead, take a pen and paper and ask yourself the following questions: Are you planning to develop a DIY product for your oily or dry skin? Are you looking for a

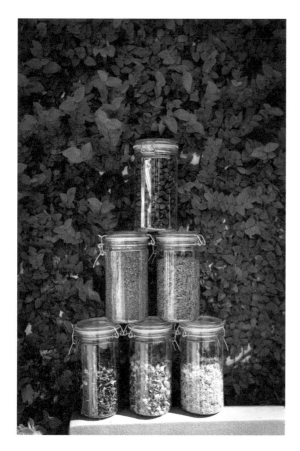

cream-based product or water-based? Do you like a floral theme or woodsy? If you plan to create an oil cleanser for your acne-prone skin, look into lightweight oil, while dehydrated/dry skin requires a different oil!

2. Figure out the functional aspect of the product

If you are looking to make a nice body scrub, pistachio or walnut shells can serve as the main functional ingredient that will exfoliate the body, while salt/sugar/oil serve as the product's base. Likewise, if you are looking to

make a hydrating face mask, you should know which ingredient will provide hydration to your skin (e.g., honey or glycerin). If you are into aromatherapy facial steam, it's essential to add aromatic herbs/peels into the formula.

3. Measure ingredients by weight

Using weight-based measurements will help you achieve more desirable results with your homemade beauty recipes. When making a small quantity, it might be okay to measure in cups and spoons, but when making large quantities or batches, it becomes tricky, and you might not always get the same end product. You will also find that measurements vary by form. For example, you can find cocoa butter in wafers, bars, or flakes. If you measure all these forms using spoons and cups, it won't give you the right measurement. These different forms of butter might take up more or less space, affecting the overall amount used in your recipes. So, instead of cups/spoons, the weight-based formula is the way to go.

How to Calculate Any DIY Recipe

1. First, decide on the total weight of the product you want to make. For example, let's say you want to make 50 ounces/50 milliliters of chocolate almond facial cream.

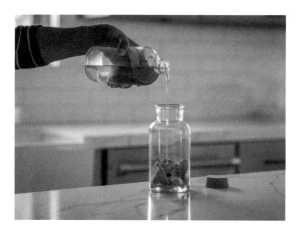

2. Gather all necessary ingredients such as cocoa butter, carrot peel–infused almond oils, and vitamin E.

3. Let's say we need 20 ounces of cream made from cocoa butter. The formula would be 20 (ounces) multiplied by 100, then divided by 50. Two thousand divided by 50 equals 40, which equals the percentage of cocoa butter we would use for facial cream.

4. Now, let's calculate the rest of the ingredients. Generally, vitamin E shouldn't be more than 1–2 percent of the formula, as it acts as an antioxidant, and we don't need it in a higher quantity. Vitamin E also protects the oil from going rancid.

5. Next, your DIY recipe formula should always add up to 100 percent. For this example, you would use 40 percent cocoa butter, 1 percent vitamin E, and the rest, 59 percent, carrot peel–infused almond oil.

6. Finally, when you're creating your product, it's important to make sure that you add the ingredients in the right order. This book's recipes divide the ingredients into "phases" so that you can easily see which ones need to be added first. This is especially important for oil- and water-based ingredients, which need to be added at different times in the skin-care product process. By following the phases listed in the book, you can be sure that all of the ingredients are added in the right order and that nothing gets missed.

This whole process takes time and practice, so having a small journal for this self-care ritual can be helpful. Write it down! I enjoy it and believe it to be the best way to document your sustainable beauty journey.

Now that we have gone through the step-by-step process of designing DIY skincare products, let's go over some basic roles that natural ingredients play in DIY skincare recipes. Before you embark on your DIY journey, get familiar with the following ingredients.

Base/Foundational Ingredients

The following ingredients make up a significant portion of the recipes in this book:

plant-based carrier oils, butters and waxes, hydrosols, water, and Dr. Bronner's Pure-Castile Soap.

Plant-Based Carrier Oils

Carrier oils serve as the base for many recipes in this book, whether you use them as is or mix them with dried fruit peels or stems. Carrier oils are derived from the fatty portion of plants, such as seeds or kernels. Here, we are taking sustainability one step further and adding food scraps along with carrier oils. Carrier oils contain several benefits for your hair and skin, and you can apply them directly.

I have a solid cultural bond regarding carrier oils that goes back to Indian winters and my mom applying these oils all over her body in the cold mornings. My mom still uses different carrier oils for her daily skin-care rituals, and I can see how her skin is still well moisturized and supple at her age. I inherited many of her beauty habits, particularly applying carrier oils to my hair, body, and face daily.

After studying at Formula Botanica, I learned a robust way to convert carrier oils into the best facial and body serums in the most affordable way. For example, whenever I feel that my hair is not soft enough or is getting dry, I apply a mixture of pure amla oil and good old castor oil before I wash my hair. The result is smoother and silkier hair.

In ancient Vedic literature and Ayurveda (an alternative medicine system), oil massages are considered a vital wellness ritual. In Indian culture, even newborn babies get coconut oil massages from their grandmas. I would like to share more knowledge about carrier oils here, so let's dig in!

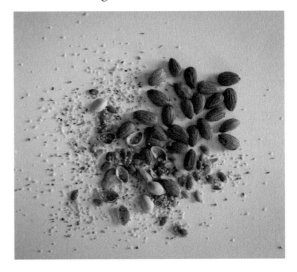

All about Carrier Oils

In natural skin care, carrier oils are popular as base oils because they are often anhydrous (water-free). These products include body butter, lip balms, cleansing balms, salves, and more. Carrier oils are by-products derived from the nuts or seeds of a plant. Since they are derived from the purest sources, and the basic chemistry of the natural source remains the same, I consider them potent, sustainable, and clean beauty products. You will see two types of carrier oils on the market: unrefined (virgin, cold-pressed) and refined.

So, what is the difference between unrefined oil and refined oil? Unrefined oil is the purest form of natural ingredient. It is minimally processed and retains more active compounds, while refined oil is further processed.

There are two methods of processing oils from nuts and seeds: cold-pressing and heated extraction. The raw process is carried out in cold-pressing at 80–90°F (yes, it is considered cold for this process!). The heated extraction method, also known as expeller pressing, is performed through mechanical machinery at approximately 120–200°F.

Unrefined oils have a slightly shorter shelf life than refined oils due to more active compounds, but I still prefer to use the unrefined version whenever I make my DIY skin-care products. There are two reasons for this: It is the purest form and contains active compounds that benefit personal wellness and skincare, and when made in smaller quantities its shelf life is not as essential.

Chemistry of Carrier Oils

Any carrier oil will contain tons of fatty acids (oleic acid, palmitoleic acid), minerals, vitamin E, phytosterols, and many more. Our skin and hair need these fatty acids. A carrier oil's chemical structure determines the physical characteristics of that particular oil. These characteristics include being hard (oil is solid at room temperature) or soft (oil remains liquid at room temperature). Oils can also have the qualities of fast absorption, slow absorption, and the list goes on. These basic terminologies will help us when we buy these oils.

There are three ways oils can be incorporated into a skin-care product:

1. Carrier oils/base oils
Carrier oils are vegetable oils such as coconut oil, avocado oil, sweet almond oil, or apricot kernel oil. These are the mainstream carrier oils, but the choices are endless.

2. Infused oils
Infused oils are also known as oil macerations, in which various botanicals are submerged into the base/carrier oil for an extended period of time. During the infusion process, natural plant compounds and carrier oil compounds are slowly processed into each other, imparting botanical benefits to the oils. Sometimes the finished oil retains the pleasant fragrance and color of the botanicals. The infused oil can be applied directly to your skin, as it is still considered a pure base oil with a botanical quality.

3. Essential oils
Essential oils are made from a well-defined process. They contain intense aromas and therapeutic values. Never apply essential oils directly to your skin, as they are potent and contain sensitizers that can irritate your skin.

Benefits of Commonly Used Carrier Oils

Sweet almond oil:

This oil contains an abundance of vitamin A, which helps soothe the redness and irritation of your skin. It's the best oil for developing under-eye recipes. Although you will find many almond oils in the market, unrefined, cold-pressed, organic is the best for home-made beauty products. It is also affordable and easy to get from most natural grocery stores. Store almond oil in the original container at a temperature of 50°F (10°C–12°C) in a cool, dark place.

Castor oil:

While this sticky oil is not a popular carrier oil for infusions, it can be a great addition when your skin needs extra softening. It helps retain moisture from the skin, which gives you supple skin. Due to its thick consistency, this oil also provides fab shine to your hair.

Apricot kernel oil:

This oil contains essential fatty acids and vitamin A. It's one of my favorites because it's fast absorbing, so it makes an ideal choice for oily/acne-prone skin. It's also an ideal choice for antiaging recipes.

Avocado oil:

Besides its usefulness in preparing meals, avocado oil has incredible benefits for the skin. It has antioxidants and anti-inflammatory properties to help your skin stay smooth, firm, and elastic. It can be applied to the body directly or mixed with other beauty products, peels, or stems. When dealing with dry skin, avocado oil can be your hero ingredient.

Coconut oil:

Coconut oil is an Indian gem here to stay. Growing up in India, I still remember my mom suggesting coconut oil as a solution for all skin- and hair-problems. Nowadays, the beauty market is saturated with numerous coconut oil products, and for good reason! Coconut oil is a great option for an overnight hair mask, as it promotes healthy hair growth, reduces hair loss, and prevents sun damage.

Olive oil:

Olive oil is likely a staple in your kitchen pantry, but it can also work wonders on the skin when used topically. If you are the owner of dry/dehydrated and compromised skin, a simple olive oil might be a great candidate to reach for during winter. It promotes collagen production and helps your skin retain moisture.

Sunflower oil:

This oil is the perfect lightweight carrier oil, promoting healthy balance regardless of skin type. It contains linolic acid, oleic acid, and vitamin E. Sunflower oil is also noncomedogenic, meaning it will not clog your pores or irritate your skin. You can get this oil from your grocery store.

Argan oil:

Argan oil is extracted from the core of the argan tree and is one of the more popular carrier oils, as it is a good source of antioxidants and vitamins. This lightweight oil moisturizes your skin and hair.

Grapeseed oil:

Grapeseed oil is actually a by-product of the winemaking industry. Once the grapes are squeezed for wine, the seeds contain amazing grapeseed oil. This oil has high levels of linoleic acid, a fatty acid that can control acne by unclogging pores, and anti-inflammatory and anti-microbial properties. I adore this oil because it protects free radicals and balances skin.

Jojoba oil:

Jojoba is a liquid wax. That makes this oil suitable for the skin regardless of one's age. It works on the skin slowly and brings about the desired result. It also offers a nonstick or oily feel in lubricating and protecting the body.

Rosehip oil:

If you're looking for an oil that does it all, look no further than rosehip oil. This skin savior is great for both oily and mature skin types. It's easily absorbed into the skin, delivering a dose of hydration without clogging pores. Rosehip oil is also high in essential fatty acids, which help nourish and repair the skin's barrier. In addition, this oil is packed with antioxidants and vitamins that can help brighten the skin and improve overall radiance. So, whether you want to achieve a dewy glow or simply keep your skin healthy and hydrated, rosehip oil is a great option.

Neem oil:

For those in the know, neem oil is an ayurvedic powerhouse. This natural oil has been used in Indian skin care for centuries, and it's time the rest of the world caught on! Neem oil is rich in antioxidants, which makes it great for helping to reduce the appearance of wrinkles and fine lines. It's also effective in treating acne, as it helps to unclog pores and control sebum production. In addition, neem oil is a natural antibacterial agent, so it's great for keeping your skin clear and free of blemishes. If you're looking for a natural way to improve your skin health, look no further than neem oil!

Pomegranate seed oil:

Pomegranate seed oil is quickly becoming a popular base for DIY skin-care products. High in antioxidants and vitamins, it nourishes and protects the skin. And best of all, it is a by-product of the pomegranate industry, so it is eco-friendly and sustainable. Whether you're looking for a natural alternative to store-bought skin-care products or just want to save money by making your own, pomegranate seed oil is a great choice. You may be surprised by how easy it is to make your own luxurious skin-care products at home.

Butters and Waxes

Butters and waxes are perfect for creating a balm, lotion, or cream texture that doesn't consist of water and/or emulsifiers (an ingredient that helps mix water and oil). When I started my DIY skin-care journey, I loved working with textures by changing ratios of butter to oil to make balms, butters, creams, and lotions! Opting in unrefined and organic options always give us the desired result with no negative side effects. Here are a few of my favorite ingredients:

Cocoa butter:

Cocoa butter is not just an ingredient in tea and chocolates. It is also an effective skin-care product that softens, protects, and nourishes the skin. It is rich in antioxidants that prevent disease and damage to body cells. Its ability to moisturize the skin makes it possible to prevent stretch marks and promote skin elasticity. Cocoa butter is a homemade beauty product you should try out if you are just starting your skin-care journey.

Shea butter:

Shea butter, like coconut oil, is soothing for the skin and works well as a conditioning agent for the hair. It contains omega-6 essential fatty acids, vitamins A and E, and anti-inflammatory properties. Shea butter also contains phytosterols, which help stimulate cell growth. The importance of shea butter cannot be overemphasized. It is useful for body cream, foot cream, lip balm, and hair cream. You can get shea butter as refined (white in color) and unrefined (butter/gold colored with a fresh, nutty scent); both are useful for beauty purposes. Shea butter should be stored in a cool, dry place at a temperature of 50°F–54°F (10°C–12°C). It has a shelf life of two years.

Beeswax:

If you are not vegan, beeswax may be a great ingredient to use for balms and lip stains because it provides extra nourishment. Beeswax is available as pellets and in sheets, and can be bleached (light but not white in color) or unbleached (warm honey/yellow in color). Its melting point is 144°F (62°C) and it has a long shelf life if it is properly stored in a dark, airtight container at a temperature of 59°F–72°F (15°C–22°C).

Vegan wax:

Beeswax can be replaced with the following vegan waxes: candelilla wax (my personal favorite) and carnauba wax. Compared to other plant-based waxes, candelilla comes closest to beeswax in properties. It comes from the leaves of the candelilla shrub, which is harvested by boiling the leaves, then skimming off the wax that floats to the top. The melting point of candelilla wax is 158ºF (70ºC). It should be stored in an airtight container at a temperature of 59°F–72°F (15°C–22°C). Carnauba wax is derived from the leaves of the Copernicia prunifera tree, which is native to Brazil. Carnauba wax is often used in solid formulas, such as vegan candles and vegan lip balms. It has a high melting point, so it's ideal for products that need to withstand higher temperatures. Carnauba wax is also nontoxic, hypoallergenic, and biodegradable. These factors make it a great choice for making vegan beauty products. Other vegan waxes include soy wax, rice bran wax, rose wax, green tea wax, etc. Vegan wax can replace beeswax in most recipes but it's important to note that vegan wax often has a higher melting point than beeswax.

Mango butter:

Mango butter is a great choice for all skin types, as it helps to hydrate and retain the skin's moisture, which makes it a popular ingredient in skin-care products. Plus, mango butter is made naturally from mango seeds.

Murumuru butter:

This exotic Amazonian butter originates from the fatty part of a Muru tree. Its nourishment is extracted from the fatty part of the tree seed. Murumuru butter is known for its high omega-9 fatty acids, making it a great choice to include in foot creams, cleansing balms, and other treatments. This butter is also emollient and glossy, providing a healthy sheen to the skin or hair.

Cupuacu butter:

This Amazonian butter is a rich and creamy butter extracted from the Cupuacu tree's fruit. It's known for its emollient properties, which help keep the skin soft and hydrated. It's also rich in fatty acids, which help nourish and protect the skin.

Kokum butter:

Kokum butter is a powerhouse for skincare. This butter is made from seeds called "kokum." It can go deep into the skin and provide maximum hydration to your skin layers. Its noncomedogenic in nature, meaning it won't clog your pores.

Hydrosols

Hydrosols or floral waters are a great way to enjoy the benefits of plants without having to worry about the potency of essential oils. They can be used directly on the skin and hair and in fragrance products. I recommend buying prepreserved hydrosols, as they are water-based and will go bad if you don't use adequate preservatives alongside them. Let's look at a few types of floral waters:

Rose water:

My all-time favorite hydrosol is rose water. It has many benefits, including repairing skin damage, reducing inflammation and redness, fighting acne, and hydrating the skin. It's been used in India for centuries for its therapeutic properties and is now gaining popularity all over the world.

Lavender hydrosol:

Lavender floral water doesn't just smell great, it also has fabulous skin-care benefits! It's perfect for calming and refreshing the skin, making it a must-have for any beauty routine.

Orange blossom hydrosol:

The sweet and floral aroma of orange blossom is refreshing and uplifting. Orange blossom hydrosol is excellent for all skin types but is especially beneficial for dry or mature skin. It helps promote collagen production while providing antioxidant protection. Orange blossom hydrosol also has anti-inflammatory properties, making it ideal for sensitive skin.

Witch hazel:

This ingredient is a popular natural remedy for a variety of skin conditions. Its astringent properties make it an effective facial toner, and it can also help heal bruises, cuts, and other wounds. Witch hazel is anti-inflammatory and antibacterial, making it effective in the treatment of acne and other skin conditions. You can find witch hazel in many beauty products or use the pure extract from the plant. If you're looking for a natural way to improve your skin health, witch hazel is definitely worth trying.

Essential Oils 101

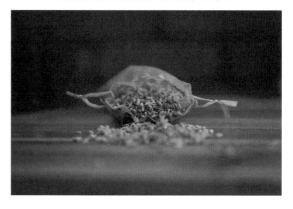

Essential oils, especially their use in cosmetics, are a controversial topic. Many beauty bloggers and experts shy away from it but I intend to provide an understanding of sustainable, transparent, and affordable skin-care products using natural ingredients before we start.

Certain cosmetic regulations expect beauty brands to comply with the International Fragrance Association (IFRA) guidelines. The IFRA represents the collective interest of the fragrance industry and has created voluntary standards for using fragrance materials. Essential oils are regulated because they contain chemical compounds that can cause a skin reaction. There are three skin reactions you can get if essential oils are not used in the proper amount: irritation, sensitization, and phototoxicity. The IFRA standards are updated every few years and they give us a clear path in terms of how many essential oils we should use in our beauty recipes and which ones are safe for our skin.

Another point to consider is the conservation status of the plant from which essential oils are obtained. Many trees are coming under increased ecological threat from the cosmetics industry (and others), leading to unsustainable beauty practices and products. Even if you make your recipes in small amounts, it is still important to be aware of this. For example, in my turmeric soap, I use a local fragrance oil instead of sandalwood because the sandalwood species is being threatened by overexploitation and regulated in its native India. The Indian government has even placed a ban on the export of timber.

Here are some other helpful tips I learned in one of the aromatherapy workshops I took a couple years ago!

1. Know your scent categories
Before mixing up an essential oil blend, consider which aromas you like the most. I have categorized essential oil aromas into five types:

- **Citrus:** If you like citrus flavors, consider using grapefruit, lemongrass, lemon, sweet orange peel (I use them in my product formulas a lot), or bergamot
- **Woodsy:** Sandalwood, frankincense, juniper, vetiver, or pine
- **Floral:** Rose, lavender, chamomile, jasmine, or ylang-ylang
- **Spicy:** Clove bud, tulsi, thyme, ginger, or turmeric
- **Oriental:** Peppermint, eucalyptus, rosemary, etc.

2. Understand notes of essential oils
Think of essential oil aromas as a musical instrument with these three notes:

- **Top notes:** Essential oils are primarily used as scents. This is the most important note to consider when formulating perfume at home. Top notes consist of small, light molecules that evaporate quickly.
- **Middle notes:** These are the heart of the scent. They perform as the main body of a perfume. These notes become a shield of base notes and cover any unpleasant aroma of base essential oils.
- **Base notes:** The base and middle notes work together to develop the central

theme of a scent. Base notes bring depth and solidity to a perfume.

3. Choose a carrier oil

I do not recommend using essential oils directly on the skin, as they are potent substances that penetrate the skin's layer, so choosing a carrier oil is necessary. I prefer jojoba oil, grapeseed oil, and fractionated coconut oil, especially during oil preparations. All of these are nongreasy with minimal fragrance and are easy to find in store. These oils will let essential oils shine.

Now that we have some basic knowledge of essential oils, let's get into the oils themselves:

Sweet orange essential oil:

Probably the happiest essential oil is my all-time favorite, sweet orange. It consists of a wonderfully uplifting and calming scent. That's why I call it a happy oil! When diffused, it can help with nervous tension and sadness and improve the aroma of your bathroom. Sweet orange oil is also antibacterial and antiviral. It is a natural detoxifier and digestive aid, cleaning out toxins and your digestive tract. It also stimulates your immune system, making it a helpful oil to have in winter.

- **Effects:** Treats acne and provide freshness to the body.

- **Uses:** Add to a diffuser for an uplifting scent or apply on your skin (dilute with a carrier oil such as coconut oil, almond oil, jojoba oil, olive oil, or avocado oil) for some much-needed relaxation.
- **Main constituent:** Limonene.
- **Aroma:** Juicy-fresh, light citrus scent.
- **Plant part:** Fruit peel.

Lavender essential oil:

If you are feeling down, stressed, and anxious, or are looking for ways to brighten up your day, try lavender essential oil. Lavender oil has been used and cherished for centuries for its unmistakable aroma and myriad benefits. In ancient times, the Egyptians and Romans used lavender for bathing, relaxation, cooking, and as a perfume. When taken internally, its calming and relaxing qualities continue to be lavender's most notable attributes. Lavender oil is frequently used to reduce the appearance of skin imperfections. Add to bath water to soak away stress. Add a few drops of lavender oil to pillows or bedding to relax and prepare for a restful night's sleep. Due to lavender's versatile properties, it is considered a must-have oil to have on hand.

- **Effects:** Eases anger/sadness and boosts your self-esteem. If you are having difficulty sleeping at night, this will help you. It can also be used for lowering high blood pressure and boosting the nervous system, and it works great when you added to a diffuser.

- **Uses:** Add a few drops to your next bath or mix 1 to 2 drops of lavender essential with fractionated coconut oil and use as natural perfume. Not recommended for internal use.
- **Main constituents:** Linalool, linalyl acetate, and ocimene.
- **Aroma:** Powdery, floral, and light.
- **Plant part:** Flower.

Rose absolute:

Rose absolute is high in a constituent called phenylethyl alcohol (PEA) which separates from the oil when steam distilled. I don't use this ingredient directly on my skin, but I like to massage a few herbs with 2 drops of rose before making products like massage oils and facial serums. The difference between absolutes and essential oils is the method of obtaining the oil. Absolutes are obtained through solvent extraction. A solvent can be a chemical or alcohol. In solvent extraction, a solvent is combined with plant material. The solvent attracts the oil from the plant material, separating the solvent from the oil. This process makes absolutes more concentrated than essential oils.

- **Effects:** Balances hormones, relieves stress, and improves circulation.
- **Uses:** Add a drop of absolute to your rinse-off products to minimize wrinkles, mix rose absolute and olive oil to improve skin suppleness, add 1 to 2 drops to your shampoo or conditioner for a delicious scent, or try making DIY potpourri for a pleasant aroma.
- **Main constituents:** Linalool, d-limonene, and benzaldehyde.
- **Aroma:** Rich, sweet, and flowery; a true rose aroma.
- **Plant part:** Flower petals.

Tea tree essential oil:

This favorite essential oil for hair is effective for treating the skin, nails, and hair and can also act as a deodorant and a mouthwash. It is an excellent choice when making bug repellent balm or lotion. Tea tree oil can treat skin conditions or improve the overall appearance of your skin if used directly to the skin because it soothes and helps heal the skin from a wide range of skin problems. Do not use it on the eye. It can cause redness and irritation. Tea tree essential oils are easily available in grocery stores or in your local pharmacy.

- **Effects:** Great cleansing properties, effectively neutralizes body odors, antibacterial, and antiseptic.

- **Uses:** Add a few drops to rice flour or arrowroot powder, mix, and use it as a dry shampoo.
- **Main constituents:** Terpinen-4-ol, gamma-terpinene, and alpha-terpinene.
- **Aroma:** Fresh, woodsy, and earthy.
- **Plant part:** Leaves.

Jasmine absolute:

Known as the Queen of Essences, jasmine oil is a middle note with a long history in perfumery. It takes approximately 2,000 pounds of jasmine flowers to produce 1 pound of oil. This oil will darken with age. Its warm and intoxicating floral aroma blends well with coriander, orange, rose, or sandalwood.

- **Effects:** Prevents hair loss, balances skin tones, ultra-nourishing, and hydrating.
- **Uses:** Make 100 percent natural perfume by adding 5 drops to 10 milliliters of almond oil. Store in a roller bottle and apply as a perfume.
- **Main constituents:** Linalool and benzyl acetate.
- **Aroma:** Warm and intoxicating floral aroma.
- **Plant part:** Flowers (harvested before dawn).

Other Additive and Utilitarian Ingredients

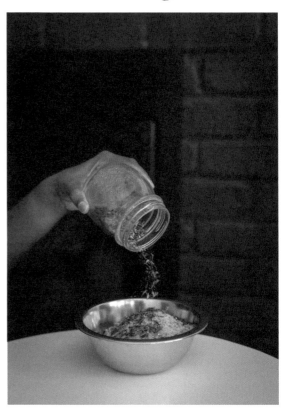

Some additive or utilitarian ingredients are necessary to make your DIY recipes the same quality as store-bought ones. For example, if you are making facial toner, you need to have water-based ingredients like hydrosols handy. In this section, I will talk about some of these basic ingredients.

Castile soap:

Castile soap is a popular base for DIY skin-care products. It's made from natural ingredients like coconut, jojoba, hemp, and palm kernel, so it's gentle on the skin and doesn't dry it out like some commercial soaps can. It's also very versatile—you can use it to make facial wash, shampoo, body wash, and more. And because it has no synthetic fragrances or chemicals, it's perfect for people with sensitive skin. If you're looking for a natural, eco-friendly, and affordable soap base, castile soap is a great choice.

Glycerin for glycerites:

Glycerin is a humectant, meaning it helps to retain moisture. This makes it great for products like shampoo, conditioner, and body wash, which can often dry out our skin. Glycerin also has a thickening effect, making it ideal for formulas that need to be thicker in consistency. We will use glycerin and dried/fresh food scraps to make a more potent base for our DIY recipes.

Vodka for tinctures:

Tinctures are a great way to enjoy the benefits of plants without having to deal with the taste or smell. Alcohol is a terrific solvent and does a better job extracting the plant's active ingredients than water does. Vodka is a good choice for making tinctures because it is relatively flavorless and has a high alcohol content. Tinctures are easy to make at home and can be taken in small doses, so they're perfect for those who want to use plants medicinally but don't want to commit to a large dose. Tinctures can be used topically or internally and added to food or drinks. When used wisely, tinctures can be a powerful ally in your quest for optimal health.

Honey:

Honey has long been a natural remedy for various ailments, but this sweet substance can also do wonders for your skin. Honey is a natural humectant, which means it helps to retain moisture. This makes it an excellent choice for people with dry or sensitive skin, as it can help keep the skin hydrated and prevent irritation. In addition, honey is easily accessible and inexpensive, making it a great option for budget-conscious skin-care enthusiasts. So, if you're looking for a natural way to improve your skin, don't be afraid to reach for the honey jar.

Vinegar for tinctures and extracts:

Vinegar is the basis for many herbal tinctures or cosmetics, and it has been a health tonic for centuries! The type I recommend for cosmetic use would have an acetic acid content of between 4%–5%; distilled white vinegars of this nature are easy to find at your grocery store. Making herbal tinctures with vinegar is an easy and inexpensive way to control every component of your cosmetic products.

Clays

Clay is a waterless ingredient that can absorb impurities from your skin, making it a fantastic cleanser. It also has anti-inflammatory and antiseptic properties. Clay serves as a refresher for your skin and can improve skin tones. When I use clay masks in my weekly skin-care rituals, I feel more vibrant, and I observe less acne and brighter, more balanced skin.

Uses of Various Types of Clay

Clay is a spa ingredient, but it can also act as a first-aid or therapeutic ingredient. In India, as per my experience, mud and water are combined to make a foot mask to remove excess heat from your body. Clay can also be a soothing agent for heat rashes, poison ivy rashes, mosquito bites, and bee stings. It works wonders when you need quick relief in an affected area. Besides its therapeutic properties, the beauty industry also uses clay masks to cure blackheads and clogged pores and to improve dull complexions.

Let's dive into the different types of clay:

Multani mitti, aka fuller's earth:

In India, ayurvedic principles are widely used in skin-care routines. One of the most popular ayurvedic ingredients is Multani mitti, a type of bleaching clay. This clay is said to have numerous benefits for the skin, including reducing the appearance of blemishes, acne scars, and blackheads. It is also said to deeply cleanse the pores, leaving the skin feeling refreshed and glowing. Some people even use Multani mitti as a face mask, allowing the clay to sit on the skin for twenty minutes or more before washing it off. While there is no scientific evidence to support these claims, many people swear by the efficacy of Multani mitti clay. If you're looking for a natural way to improve your skin's appearance, give Multani mitti, aka fuller's earth, a try!

Rhassoul clay:

Rhassoul clay is an exceptional clay with multiple benefits. It is mined in the fertile Atlas Mountains of Morocco and has been used for more than twelve centuries by North African, Southern Europe, and Middle Eastern populations. This clay is rich in silica, potassium, magnesium, and calcium. Rhassoul clay can be a hair-care product to cleanse hair and remove excess oils. It can also be a skin-care product to help improve skin elasticity and firmness. Additionally, this clay can make soaps, dry shampoos, hair scalp scrubs, and shampoos, as it has surfactant quality. Rhassoul clay is truly a versatile and beneficial product.

Kaolin clay:

I call kaolin clay a base clay. It is a gentle clay, making it a perfect sustainable ingredient for your weekly skin-care ritual. According to Ayurveda, we have skin problems because our skin pores get clogged with toxins. When our pores are clogged, it prevents our skin from breathing and functioning properly. That's where kaolin clay comes in. It helps to detoxify and stimulate your skin by drawing out impurities and stimulating circulation. Your skin will be left feeling refreshed, radiant, and balanced. So, if you're looking for a gentle yet effective way to care for your skin, add kaolin clay to your skin-care routine!

Bentonite clay:

Bentonite clay is a great option if you're looking for a natural way to detox your body and improve your skin health. This clay comprises tiny particles that act like a magnet, attracting and absorbing impurities from the body. When paired with vinegar, bentonite clay can help remove dead skin cells, reduce inflammation, and tighten pores. Your skin will feel softer and more radiant. In addition, regular use of bentonite clay can help detoxify the body and boost overall health. Bentonite clay is a great choice if you're looking for a simple way to improve your health and appearance.

French green clay:

If you've ever been to a spa, you've probably experienced the power of French green clay. This clay is commonly used in facial treatments due to its ability to absorb oils, toxins, and impurities from the skin. It also has a toning effect that can help improve the skin's overall appearance. If you're struggling with occasional blemishes, French green clay can be a helpful solution. Simply apply it to trouble spots daily or use it as a weekly facial routine. You'll soon see a noticeable difference in your skin's appearance.

Aloe vera:

Aloe vera has been used for hair care, skin care, and as a wellness product for centuries. The plant is easy to take care of and can be easily grown at home. Aloe vera gel can be used on the hair, scalp, and skin. It is a highly effective hair conditioner that can help control dandruff and hair loss and promote growth. The gel can also be used on the face and body to soothe sunburns, scars, and other skin conditions. In Ayurveda, aloe vera is considered a tridoshic herb, meaning it balances all three doshas (aka nature of the body type, which indicates your skin type as well) in the body. Whether you are looking for a natural hair conditioner or digestive aid, aloe vera is a versatile plant that can offer many benefits. If you have a green thumb, I suggest planting this goodie.

Although I have provided you with a big list of ingredients in this chapter, I strongly suggest buying them slowly or on an as-needed basis. My teachers at Formula Botanica taught me to use the KISS method whenever I am in the mood to develop my own beauty products: Keep It Simple and Short. Basically, buy only five to ten ingredients in the smallest quantity possible and try out two to three recipes at a time. Change your beauty habits slowly; that's the most sustainable and green way to change.

Patch Test

As beauty enthusiasts, we always look for the latest and greatest products to add to our routines, but before slathering new products all over our faces, it's important to do a patch test first to sense check that our skin doesn't react negatively to a new product. While this is unlikely, it's always better to be safe than sorry. Simply apply a little of the product to an inconspicuous area of skin, like your elbow or ankle, and wait twenty-four hours to see if there's any reaction. If everything looks good, continue to use the product as normal. Next time you're tempted to try out that new serum or face mask, remember to patch test first!

Chapter 3

Best Manufacturing Practices for Healthy Beauty Recipes

The best way to ensure a successful outcome when making your own DIY skin-care recipes is to follow best manufacturing practices. Best manufacturing practices involve using dedicated tools and containers, suitable raw materials and ingredients, and clean work areas and tools. Following these simple guidelines, you can avoid problems and produce safe, high-quality products.

Let me share a simple analogy to understand the importance of best manufacturing practices. As an Indian, I always have my spice box handy because that's the easiest and fastest way to make any Indian curry in no time! For this purpose, I use clean, dry containers. Having a dedicated container for this practice helps me create the same sort of taste in all my food! Similar to my spice box, I recommend creating a beauty box specifically for your DIY beauty recipes.

When it comes to DIY beauty products, one of the major things you need to understand is hygiene. Nobody wants a beauty disaster, so it's important to make sure that your recipes are as bacteria-free as possible.

Always wash your hands thoroughly, use clean utensils, and follow the recipe to the letter. Don't try to shortcut any of the steps because you'll only be compromising the final product. It's also important to use fresh ingredients and to avoid leaving products open or exposed to the elements. With skin care, it's always better to be safe than sorry!

DIY Recipes and Simple Rules

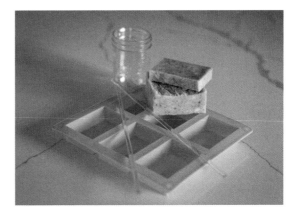

To ensure that your DIY recipes are safe, I recommend using dedicated tools and containers for each project. Keep everything in good condition by following these simple rules:

1. Only choose materials that say they're usable together; if you're not sure about the quality of an ingredient or a container, don't use it!
2. Store raw ingredients and packaged products according to package instructions (especially oils, butters, waxes, hydrosols, etc.). Be careful when handling fragile and dangerous items like alcohol tinctures or essential oils. If not used properly, they could cause problems on your skin.
3. Clean work surfaces every time you finish making a recipe. Use your kitchen essentials to make sure you're not risking any germs. Please be aware that they may have been used on somebody else's skin, so wash them in boiling water between uses or put them in the dishwasher on a sterilize cycle.
4. Note down every single step when you try any recipe for the first time. It's good to note down observations!
5. You can reuse your old containers but ensure that they are clean and dry before reusing. Using a container with still water will cause bacteria growth!
6. Invest in a good hairnet, kitchen apron, and pair of disposable gloves. These may not be essential if you're making a quick face scrub for your spa party, but they're still worth having on hand.
7. Planning out your batch size will help you calculate percentages for each ingredient with ease; deciding what material or ingredients to work with also comes down to this step. For example, if your recipe calls for infused oil, you should know that the infusion process needs to be done first!

Spending more time on paper before getting into gear saves both money (because less waste) *and* precious energy during production hours. Let's be as sustainable as we can! Come up with five types of carrier oils, two to three hydrosols, castile soap, and glycerin. Combine these ingredients with discarded food scraps and enjoy the recipe process. In a nutshell, have fun with it. Sustainable change can be hard at first, but once you know the basics, it will be a smooth ride.

Before moving further, let's talk about two chemistry rules that we need to consider when following best manufacturing practices: Why we should be careful with water, and combining water and oil.

Why We Should Be Careful with Water

Beauty and wellness manufacturers often heavily dilute their products while we remain none the wiser. Our only indicator is that cosmetic labels read from high to low with the first ingredients listed used most and last ingredients listed used least. Our government doesn't require listings by percentage on packaging, so you can't be sure what's actually in there unless it says so directly (and sometimes even then). This makes us vulnerable when shopping for products because many brands boast about the benefits of a specific ingredient their products contain without revealing exactly why those benefits matter. The general rule is that lotion, moisturizers, and creams contain 70%–80% water. That's why the DIY recipes in this book use anhydrous formulas or botanical hydrosols.

Bacteria can grow in water-based products when not treated properly, leading to the product or your recipe growing yeast, molds, and fungi, which could cause skin sensitivities or even severe reactions for some people with allergies. When using ingredients containing water such as castile soap, aloe vera gel, or floral waters, only use in small 1-ounce quantities and store in the refrigerator.

Combining Water and Oil

If you studied chemistry in high school (fun fact about me: I studied in India, and after 10th grade, you can pick and choose your subjects. And, yes, I picked chemistry!), you know that oil and water don't mix. That's

why the beauty industry came up with an awesome-sauce ingredient that they call an "emulsifier." This ingredient helps mix water and oil together to create a cream-based texture. Based on water and oil ratios and the right emulsifier, you can make lotion, washes, foot cream, hand cream, cleansing balms, and so on. In this book, I want to teach you that this texture can be achieved through the right consistency of oil, butter, and wax without adding water.

Another important point to consider is that when you use essential oils to add fragrance to your bi-phase recipes (containing both oil and water) such as makeup remover, it is necessary to disperse essential oils in another oil, Epsom salts, or oats and combine with the main recipe. Please note that essential oils won't mix well with water or hydrosols; they will stay on top and could cause skin sensitivities so mix with water very carefully!

Equipment, Tools, and Instruments

Now that we've gone over best manufacturing practices, let's get into the types of equipment, tools, and instruments you need to start your DIY skin-care journey!

1. Aluminum foil
Aluminum foil keeps food fresh by insulating it from oxygen, moisture, heat, and bacteria

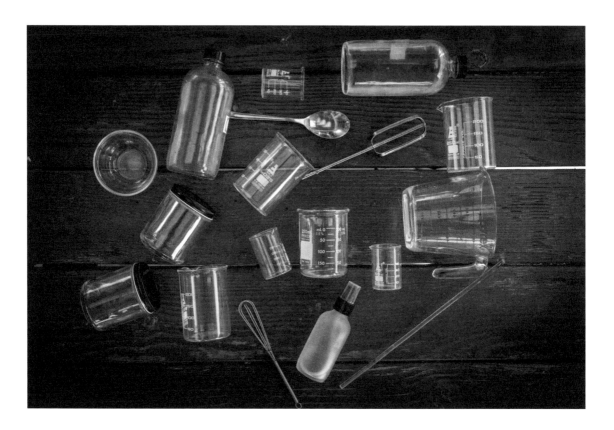

to prevent the food from going bad or taking on a smelly odor. Foil can also be used to keep the fruit peels and vegetable stems for your beauty products fresh before they are used. I strongly suggest reserving one drawer in your fridge for food scraps and labeling it for easier identification.

2. Plastic wrap

Plastic wrap is similar to aluminum foil because it has a hard barrier that protects food against bacteria and prevents food odors from spreading. The difference between aluminum foil and plastic wrap is that plastic wrap can store more acidic foods such as orange peels, lemon peels, and various fruit seeds. I love using aluminum foil and plastic wrap to store food scraps for my homemade beauty products, as they do an excellent job preserving them.

3. Airtight glass containers

Air is not ideal for food storage, especially over a long period of time. Airtight containers are useful for the peels, stems, and seeds you'll use to make homemade beauty products. They can help prevent cross-contamination when refrigerating food scraps and can also store your homemade beauty products.

4. Resealable bags (use recyclable ones and reduce your carbon footprint!)

Resealable bags are products used in the kitchen to prevent air from entering the food again. They are a compact and effective alternative to big glass containers. Resealable bags are ideal for storing food scraps that don't take up too much space such as cucumber peels and they are useful in storing homemade beauty products such as lotion bars.

5. Tin cans

The major benefit of tin cans is that they are perfect for preserving the taste and freshness of sustainable products. They can be heated to destroy harmful microorganisms and completely seal off food from air in the process, helping the food maintain its aroma and texture. In the same vein, homemade beauty products and their raw materials can be stored in tin cans; think about using tin cans to store your powdered face masks.

6. Jars, dropper bottles, and pump bottles

People who like jars should use glass jars with a metal cap. I love using jars and dropper bottles and organize them stylishly in my beauty cabinets. They provide me with the most luxurious feel. You can also reuse store-bought beauty jars after you sterilize them properly. Amber colored dropper bottles are great for storing oils because the amber color protects oils from going rancid. Pump bottles are a great choice for storing gel or face wash, as the product will not come into contact with air, leading to less contamination. I recommend keeping the following bottles on hand: 0.5-ounce, 1-ounce, 2-ounce, and 4-ounce glass jars in assorted colors (white, frosted, amber, etc.).

7. Steel funnels or recycled plastic funnels

Funnels help prevent product spillage. I recommend investing in a few sizes, as big funnels might not fit into 1-ounce or 0.5-ounce jars.

8. Cookie sheets

Cookie sheets are the way to go if you're looking for an easy way to dry out your citrus peels and stems. Just line them with parchment paper, then place your peels and stems on the sheets. Ensure that the scraps are not touching each other, then put the sheets in a cool, dry place. After a few days, your peels should be crispy and ready to use. Store them in an airtight container for up to a month. To get fancy, you can even dust them with cocoa powder or ground coffee before drying them out. Just don't eat too many; they're addictive!

9. Ice trays

An ice tray is a great way to store dried-out peels, seeds, and stems.

Kitchen Equipment Used for Beauty Products

The benefits of making your own beauty products cannot be overemphasized, as it allows you to determine what you put on (which gets absorbed *in*) your body. We live in a world where we possess many kitchen gadgets for making tasty food items, so why not make luxurious, affordable, and 100 percent natural skin- and hair-care products using those gadgets as well? Let's talk about some of the kitchen gadgets we will use throughout this book:

1. Digital kitchen scale (measure from 0.1–1 ounce)
A scale is an important first step in measuring dry, liquid, or solid ingredients. You can get away with measuring in tablespoons or cups if you're measuring dry and liquid ingredients only, but we will measure ingredients by weight in this book, so measuring in ounces is preferred. Don't bother buying a new precision scale; a good old kitchen scale will work just fine.

2. Coffee grinder
The second item on my list is another inexpensive one but it's also another important step in measuring your ingredients. I generally use a coffee grinder to grind dried food peels and seeds into powders for foam-based cleansing powders, face masks and scrubs, walnut shell powder, and shikakai (an ayurvedic herb) powder. A coffee grinder will make sure that the right quantity of ingredients grinds well with no fuss.

3. Steel or aluminum spoon sets
Wooden spoons absorb moisture which can cause bacteria down the line, so I strongly suggest investing in a good steel or aluminum metal spoon set for your recipes.

4. Mesh strainer
A mesh strainer is an important and effective kitchen item for making beauty products. See it as "quality control" for your recipes.

5. Double boiler or bain-marie
A double boiler or bain-marie is a big pot filled with water and topped with a heat-proof glass bowl for melting ingredients. This kitchen item helps melt butters, waxes, and oils more gently. If you melt them at too high of a temperature, they lose their botanical value.

6. Kitchen converter app
Use this tool to convert measurements; it is available on your smartphone. It helps do the job effortlessly, especially for those who are bad at math. It also saves time.

7. Electric blender or beater

A hand blender works just fine for most recipes, but in cases where you need control over the speed to whip those ingredients more smoothly, an electric blender or beater gives you more control. Plus, electric blenders are also easier to clean. Just throw them into the dishwasher.

8. Spatula

A spatula ensures that you get most of your product out of your blender. The shape of the spatula helps in achieving this. However, make sure you have a separate spatula for beauty products and food products. You don't want to touch your cookie dough with the same spatula used for mixing essential oils and Epsom salt!

9. Measuring spoons and mixing bowls

Even though we will not measure our ingredients in spoons and cups, measuring spoons can be beneficial when it comes to scooping out certain ingredients from the packaging (e.g., cocoa butter, shea butter, or coconut oil). Mixing bowls are another great staple to have handy when making a big batch or stirring up ingredients.

10. Hairnet and apron

A hairnet is essential, as you don't want your hair to get inside your beauty products, and an apron will protect you against spills. (And

nothing wrong in feeling something like a chemist!)

11. Food dehydrator

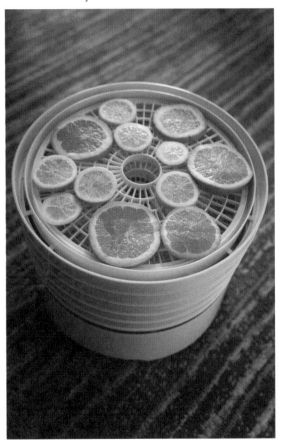

If you're the type of person who hates wasting food, a food dehydrator is a kitchen appliance you need to invest in. With a food dehydrator, drying out peels and stems of fruits and vegetables that would normally end up in the trash turns them into healthy snacks. You can even dry out herbs from your garden to make homemade herb blends. Dehydrated foods also have a longer shelf life than fresh foods, so you can cook in bulk and have healthy meals on hand when you're short on time. A food dehydrator is a kitchen appliance worth investing in if you're looking for a way to reduce food waste and eat healthier.

When I started my DIY skin-care journey, I emptied one shelf from my kitchen cabinet. Slowly, I gathered more herbs and raw ingredients, and now I have a separate lab area set up. The robust recipes included in this book will teach you how to make DIY beauty products for your own needs and skin type. In the following chapter, I will discuss commonly known facts and best ingredients for our skin.

Chapter 4
Base Formulas

The oil production and moisture content in your skin determine your skin type (oily, dry, etc.). If you've struggled to treat your skin type with store-bought beauty products, I recommend trying your own sustainable skin-care solutions instead. Let's walk through the steps of better understanding our skin.

The Anatomy of the Skin

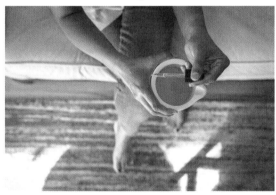

The skin is our largest organ at about twenty square feet. It protects us from microbes and the elements by shredding thirty- to forty-thousand dead cells per minute (sounds shocking, but that's what science tells us). It also regulates body temperature by adjusting insulin levels in response to food intake or exercise and permits sensations like touch (capability for pain), hot, and cold, which help maintain human life!

The skin is a self-renewing, nutrient-providing organ constructed from the foods you eat. It's important to remember that while skin-care products can help keep your complexion looking fresh and young, there's no one tool or product in this world that will make an instant transformation happen on its own! In general, our skin renewal process takes 28–45 days. When we are young, the skin renewal process is faster, but when we grow older, that renewal process takes time. In this book, my DIY beauty recipes will help the skin renewal process in a healthy way.

Our skin consists of three layers:

1. Epidermis
The epidermis or "top skin," as it is often called (because we apply products to this part first), acts like a protective barrier against external aggressors such as UV rays from sunlight or pollution particles.

2. Dermis
The dermis is a tough layer that is slightly thicker than skin. It is made up of mostly

collagen fibers surrounded by elastic fibers, which give it its strength but also allow for flexibility when needed most! The dermis is one of the most important layers of our skin. It provides nutrients for epidermal cells and houses blood vessels and nerves. The dermis can tell us if something's wrong with your body before it gets worse because this part contains warning devices such as pain, which will activate when damage occurs, so you'll know what needs attention right away.

3. Hypodermis

The hypodermis is a deep, thick layer of tissue that stores energy, insulates against heat loss, and provides cosmetic benefits for the skin. This subcutaneous tissue contains coarse bundles of collagen and fat cells called adipocytes that release energy as heat or generate hormones such as insulin, which helps control blood sugar levels for people with diabetes.

Hair follicles, nails, and sebaceous glands also play an important role in your skin's health. Hair comprises three main parts: the cortex, the medulla, and the cuticle. The cortex is the innermost layer of your hair and is made up of long, coiled proteins called keratin fibers. These fibers are arranged in a spiral pattern that give your hair its strength and flexibility. The medulla is a spongy core in the center of your hair that gives it strength and structure.

The cuticle is the outermost layer of your hair and includes long, overlapping scales that protect the inner layers of your hair from damage.

Our nails grow out from beneath the surface-level tissue near our fingers and toes called "live cuticles." It's easy for damage to occur here because we're constantly touching things with these delicate parts; however, any injuries will heal with time if left alone. Some people have weak or brittle nail beds due in part to improper diet choices (such as eating too much sugar), but more often than not, they're caused by constant activity without giving your feet some rest.

There are two types of sweat glands in the human body: eccrine and apocrine. Eccrine glands are the major source of sweat in our bodies. They help us survive hot environments like those found in an overheated house or on an airplane, keeping us cool by releasing perspiration that evaporates when exposed to air. Apocrine glands (like the ones in your armpit) secrete sweat with an odor and produce droplets bigger than other kinds, which make them smell worse!

Why Do We Need Base Recipes?

We all play many roles in our lives: student, professional, parent, etc. I totally get that adding even one more thing to your to-do list can feel like a lot, which is why my version of meal planning (but for skin care!) can help you better prioritize your skin-care routine.

Think about this scenario: If you don't meal plan for the week, it's almost certain that you will order in some nights. Even though you desire to feed yourself healthy and nutritious food, your physical energy is not always there to make dinner each and every night. The same theory applies to your skin-care routine. If you don't create base formulas ahead of time, you won't always have the energy to stir up your own beauty products each and every day. The following section will give you all the tools to create your own base formulas ahead of time for whenever you need them!

Base Formulas for DIY Recipes

A base formula for any DIY recipe consists of foundational and functional/active ingredients with aromatic, additive, and aesthetic properties. You can't make body oil without oil or toner without hydrosol or water because those ingredients are the backbone of any DIY beauty product; that's why they're called foundational ingredients. When you develop your own balms, creams, toners, oils, or lotions, you always want to make sure you use proper oil, butter, water, or wax. Functional or active botanicals are the

herbs and herbal extracts, such as macerated/infused oils (scrappy tinctures) or glycerites, that add the nourishing, moisturizing, or revitalizing power to products. Based on the maceration or infusion method, active botanical properties can be transferred into an oil or water-based medium. Additive ingredients include pigments, vitamin E, and preservatives (e.g., honey), while aromatic ingredients include essential oils or food scraps such as citrus peels to make your DIY more luxurious and therapeutic. Not all DIY products need to look aesthetically pleasing, but incorporating natural ingredients such as orange or grapefruit peels might be a good way to make your body scrubs or soaps more interesting.

Base Recipes

Now that we know the basics of a base formula, let's make our own base recipes using food scraps such as peels, shells, stems, and seeds.

Powdered Herbal Scraps

If you're like me, you hate wasting food, but no matter how hard you try, there always seem to be a few leftover scraps you just can't use up. Instead of throwing them away, why not turn them into something useful? For example, you can dry out peels and stems in a dehydrator or oven to create a healthy powdered scrap. Just grind dried scraps into a fine powder using a coffee grinder or blender, then add them to a face mask, face scrub, bath tea—anything you can think of! Not only will you be reducing food waste, but you'll also be adding extra nutrients to your skin care. Win-win! These powders can also be oven-dried, frozen, or sun-dried. See the following recipes to learn more.

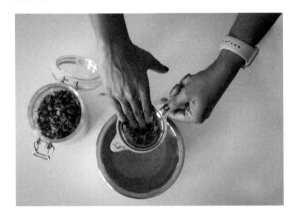

Basic recipe for oven-dried powders:
Fruit and vegetable peels can take years to biodegrade into your compost so, instead of throwing away those skin-loving nutrients which can glow your skin instantly, make this recipe out of them!

Good peels for oven-drying:
Carrot peels, orange peels, grapefruit peels, lime/lemon peels, potato peels, sweet potato peels, cucumber peels, zucchini peels, beetroot peels

Classic formula/tips for oven-dried powders:
Ingredients: 1 cup organic fruit or vegetable peels, cut into small chunks (it's not desirable to turn on your giant oven for just a few scraps so I suggest storing them in the refrigerator until you've collected at least 1 cup)

Method: Line a cookie sheet with parchment paper and preheat the oven to 170°F. Spread your scraps onto the lined cookie sheet and bake for 45 to 60 minutes. Put the peels into small airtight jars/containers and store in the refrigerator. This powdered herbal scrap can be used in oil infusions.

General shelf life: 6 months

Sample Formula

Ingredients	Percentage of Ingredients Needed
Fresh food scraps (e.g., fruit/vegetable peels, seeds)	100%

Frozen Herbal Scraps
Frozen herbal scraps are great for bath teas, foot soaks, foot scrubs, and especially scalp scrubs.

Good stems/peels to freeze:
Coriander stems, mint stems, rosemary/thyme/oregano stems, spinach/kale stems,

fennel leaves, lemon peels, lime peels, apple peels, beet root stems, banana peels

Classic formula/tips for frozen scraps:

Ingredients: A small amount of peels works well with this method.

Method: This method is perfect if you are peeling vegetables or making a salad and you know that you will throw away your vegetable stems. Instead of putting those scraps into the garbage, wash them thoroughly in cold water and add them to a resealable bag or airtight container or cut them into small pieces and add them to an ice tray. This method works well when making an eye mask or hair scalp scrub.

General shelf life: 2 months

Sample Formula

Ingredients	Percentage of Ingredients Needed
Fresh food scraps (e.g., fruit/vegetable peels, seeds)	100%

Sun-Dried Herbal Scraps

Growing up in India, I had no access to an oven or freezer during my childhood. Thus, sun-dried methods came in handy. I still remember my mom making sun-dried potato chips or rice flour papadum using this sun-dried method.

Good peels/seeds for sun-drying:

Lemon peels, lime peels, orange peels, passion fruit peels, kumquat peels, tangerine peels, mango seeds, pumpkin seeds, pomegranate peels

Classic formula/tips for sun-dried powders:

Ingredients: Lemon peels/lime peels/apple peels/beet root stems, or any food peels you have handy in your kitchen.

Method: Wash your desired food scraps well and set aside. Lay out a large tablecloth or other cotton cloth outside in the sun and add weights to the corners. Lay your food scraps on top and rotate them every other day. Once your scraps harden (this could take anywhere from a few days up to a month), store them in airtight containers or jars. Don't keep moisture anywhere near dried scraps.

General Shelf Life: 6 months

Sample Formula

Ingredients	Percentage of Ingredients Needed
Fresh food scraps (e.g., fruit/vegetable peels, seeds)	100%

Scrappy Tinctures (extracts made with alcohol/ethanol)

A scrappy tincture is an alcohol- or ethanol-based soluble medium that dissolves all the hidden goodies of food scraps. Tinctures are sometimes called concentrated herbal extracts. Alcohol tinctures are a great way to enjoy the benefits of herbal medicine without having to take the time to make an infusion. They are also more concentrated than water infusions, so you only need a small amount. Tinctures can be stored in small dropper bottles and tucked into a purse or bag, which makes them very convenient for those with busy lifestyles. In addition, tinctures are easily and quickly absorbed into the bloodstream, making them ideal for those who need quick relief.

Good peels/seeds for scrappy tinctures:
Lemon peels, lime peels, orange peels, passion fruit peels, cucumber peels, kumquat

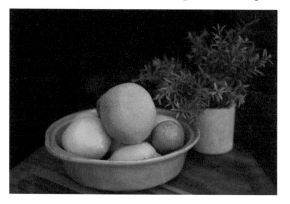

peels, tangerine peels, mango seeds, pumpkin seeds, beetroot peels, pomegranate peels

Methods/tips & tricks:

Random-measured method: You can use fresh or dried food scraps with this method. Wash and remove all dirt and food residue from fresh peels, and seeds. Chop fresh food scraps or grind/crush dried scraps with a coffee grinder. Place prepared scraps into a canning jar with a lid and add enough alcohol to submerge all scraps in the alcohol by 1 inch. If food scraps come above the alcohol level, it can cause oxidization and the entire mixture can become contaminated or moldy. Put wax paper on top of the jar before closing the lid. Store jar in a cool, dark place such as a cupboard for 4 to 6 weeks. After 4 to 6 weeks, strain the mixture through a wire strainer or cheesecloth. Pour the mixture into dark-colored glass bottles and store in a dark, cool place.

Weighted method: With this method, we generally measure one part (1 ounce) fresh food scraps and two parts (2 ounces) alcohol. If using dried food scraps, measure one part (1 ounce) dried food scraps and four parts (four ounces) alcohol.

General shelf life: 4–6 months

Sample Formula (if using fresh scraps)

Ingredients	Percentage of Ingredients Needed
Fresh food scraps (e.g., fruit/vegetable peels, seeds)	10%
Alcohol (e.g., Absolut Vodka)	90%

Sample Formula (if using dried scraps)

Ingredients	Percentage of Ingredients Needed
Dried food scraps (e.g., fruit/vegetable peels, seeds)	40%
Alcohol (e.g., Absolut Vodka)	60%

Infusions (extracts made by infusing herbs in oils or fats)

Oil infusions are all the rage these days, and for a good reason. Not only are they a great way to pamper your skin, but they can also be used for a variety of other purposes, from healing cuts and scrapes to soothing sunburns. You can also add them to homemade lotions and body butter, use them as massage oils, or apply them directly to your skin. You can even add infused oils to salad dressings or use them as a healthy alternative to butter or olive oil. With so many potential uses, oil infusions are sure become a staple in your beauty and wellness routine.

An infused oil, also called a macerated oil, contains dried herbs or food scraps. (If you use fresh scraps, you run the risk of microbiological infection and your oil could get ruined.) There are two main ways to make an oil infusion: gentle heat or rapid heat. Rapid heat infusions are generally quicker, but gentle infusions are better suited for delicate ingredients like flowers or herbs. Whichever method you choose, the basic principle is the same: infusing oil with your chosen ingredient(s) to extract their beneficial properties.

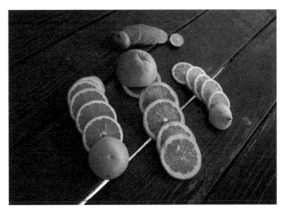

Good peels/seeds for infusions:
Lemon peels, lime peels, orange peels, passion fruit peels, cucumber peels, kumquat peels, tangerine peels, mango seeds, pumpkin seeds, beetroot peels, pomegranate peels

Methods/tips & tricks:

Gentle heat (sun-infusion method): The sun is a great source of energy for extracting herbal particles from food scraps. To use this method, place dehydrated food scraps in a canning jar and submerge the scraps in oil, making sure the scraps are totally covered with at least ½–1 inch of oil. Screw the cap on tightly and leave jars near a sunny windowsill. Leave this canning jar on a countertop and shake it daily. Do this for at least 3 to 4 weeks. After 3 to 4 weeks, strain the oil from the food scraps using a cheesecloth. Let all the oil drip out, then squeeze the scraps to extract the remaining oil. Pour this infused oil into a dark-colored jar and store it in a cool, dark place.

General shelf life: 3 months

Rapid heat (gas/stove method): This method comes in handy when you want to create a marvelous body cream or oil cleanser within a day. To start, place dehydrated food scraps into a heatproof jar and fully submerge the scraps in oil. Put this jar into a double boiler and turn the heat to the lowest temperature possible. Keep this jar in the double boiler for 4 to 6 hours and keep an eye on the stove. Alternatively, you can use a slow cooker and keep the oil mixture on a low setting for 8 hours. Strain the oil from the food scraps using a cheesecloth. Let all the oil drip out, then squeeze the scraps to extract the remaining oil. Pour this infused oil into a dark-colored jar and store it in a cool, dark place.

General shelf life: 3 months

Sample Formula

Ingredients	Proportion of Ingredients Needed
Dried food scraps (e.g., fruit/vegetable peels, seeds)	⅓ cup food scraps
Carrier oil (e.g., grapeseed oil, olive oil, apricot kernel oil, almond oil)	⅔ cup carrier oil

Glycerites (extracts made by infusing herbs or food scraps in glycerin)

Glycerin is such a versatile ingredient because it can extract all the golden nuggets that food scraps have to offer without destroying their natural properties. The best part about making glycerites? You do not need to dry your scraps first. Glycerites are also a fabulous option if you are making anything for kids, as they have no alcohol. Glycerites can be added to water-based products such as skin tonics, body washes, micellar waters, cleansers, and shampoos.

Good peels/seeds for glycerites:
Lemon peels, lime peels, orange peels, passion fruit peels, cucumber peels, kumquat

peels, tangerine peels, mango seeds, pumpkin seeds, beetroot peels, pomegranate peels

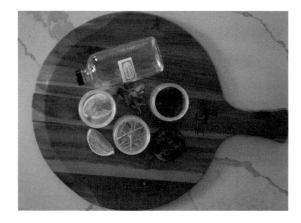

Method/tips & tricks:

It is easy to control, monitor, and develop glycerites with single ingredients. To make this base recipe more precise, I generally use a kitchen scale and try to choose organic/untreated vegetable scraps. Wash any fresh scraps thoroughly and cut them into small pieces. Put those pieces into mason jars and pour glycerin on top. The jars should be kept at room temperature away from direct sunlight and heat. Depending on the food scraps used, your glycerin infusion can be ready within 2 to 7 days.

Before straining your solution, make sure to sanitize your surroundings. Using coffee filter paper and another mason jar, strain the solution. The straining process could take anywhere from 2 to 30 minutes. Add the filtered glycerin solution to an airtight container and refrigerate.

General shelf life: 2 weeks

Sample Formula (if using fresh scraps)

Ingredients	Percentage of Ingredients Needed
Fresh food scraps (e.g., fruit/vegetable peels, seeds)	20%
Glycerin	80%

Sample Formula (if using dried scraps)

Ingredients	Percentage of Ingredients Needed
Dried food scraps (e.g., fruit/vegetable peels, seeds)	40%
Glycerin	60%

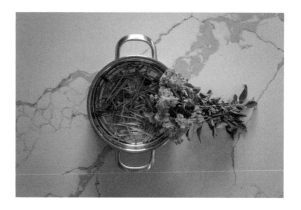

Recipes for Skin- and Hair-Care

Here are a few additional recipes to help you build your own beauty apothecary:

1. Sweet potato peel powder using oven-dried method

Did you know that sweet potato peels are great for skin? That's right—the humble sweet potato peel can help keep your skin looking young and healthy. Here's how: Sweet potato peels are packed with antiaging antioxidants. These powerful nutrients protect your skin from damage caused by harmful free radicals and prevent fine lines and wrinkles by locking in moisture, keeping your skin hydrated, and preventing dryness. So, next time you're cooking sweet potatoes, don't throw out the peels; use them to give your skin a boost instead!

Method: Use organic sweet potatoes if possible. Wash peels very thoroughly and dry with a kitchen towel to remove all dampness. Preheat the oven to 220°F. Add scraps to a parchment paper–lined cookie sheet and bake for 40 minutes. Rotate the peels throughout. Once the peels are crispy, add them to a coffee grinder. Grind until a nice fine powder is reached. Store in tin jars in a cool, dark place.

2. Carrot peel oil infusion using gentle heat method

Carrot peels are often overlooked as a skin-care ingredient, but they actually offer a wide range of benefits. For starters, carrot peels are anti-inflammatory, which can help soothe irritated skin. They're also packed with antioxidants and vitamins A, C, and E, which help protect the skin from damage and keep it looking healthy. In addition, carrot peels are hydrating and moisturizing, making them ideal for preventing dryness and keeping the skin feeling soft and supple. Next time you're peeling carrots, don't toss out the peels; your skin will thank you for it!

Method: This DIY recipe is simple and only requires a few ingredients. First, choose the oil you want to use. A light olive oil, avocado oil, or vegetable oil works well. Then, add oven-dried carrot peels to the oil. Place the mixture in a glass jar and seal it tightly. Then, set the jar in a sunny spot and let it infuse for 1 to 2 weeks. When the infusion is complete, strain out the carrot peels and store the oil in a cool, dark place. You can use this oil as a body oil, but I love to use it in my body balms, body butters, or foot scrubs. It acts as a great hair oil as well.

3. Lemon peel glycerite

Lemon peels are often used in skin-care products due to their high concentration of citric acid that helps to exfoliate the skin, remove dead skin cells, and unclog pores. Lemon peels also have a pH of 2, making them acidic enough to act as an alpha hydroxy acid (AHA). AHAs are often used in skin-care products to improve the texture of skin by reducing fine lines, wrinkles, and age spots. If you're looking to make a skin-care product with a little extra oomph, consider adding lemon peel.

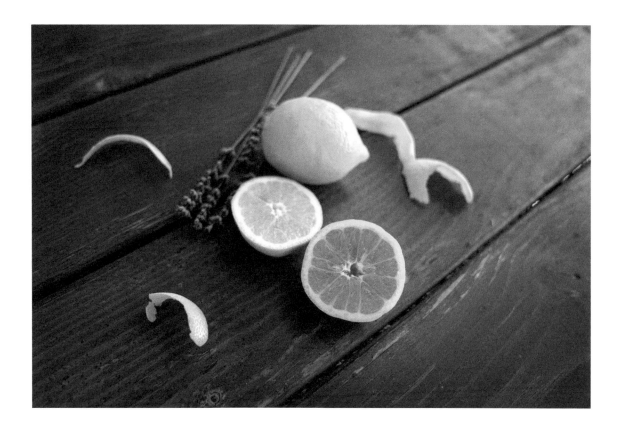

Method: First, scrub the lemon in distilled water. Then, slice and/or chop the lemon (include both peel and fruit). Weigh the lemon and the glycerin, add them to a jar with a lid, then seal. This glycerite can be used in toners, face masks, and face scrubs.

4. Pistachio shell powder

The next time you're snacking on pistachios, don't throw away the shells! These humble leftovers can be used for a variety of skin-care purposes.

Methods: They make an excellent exfoliating scrub once you grind them nicely in your coffee grinder. Add a little water and some honey to form a paste, then massage it onto your skin in a circular motion. The shells will help slough away dead skin cells, while the honey will nourish and hydrate your skin. You can also use pistachio shells to make a soothing face mask. Simply grind them into a powder and mix with some yogurt and lemon juice. Apply the mask to your face and leave it on for about 15 minutes before rinsing off. The yogurt will help calm any irritation, while the fatty acids in the pistachio shell powder will help keep your skin soft and supple. So, don't throw out those pistachio shells; put them to good use instead!

5. Orange peel tincture

If you're looking for an easy scrap to add to your home apothecary, orange peel is a great choice. You can use the peels from organically grown oranges; just save them when you're done eating the fruit.

Method: To prepare orange peels for tincturing or potpourri, shave off the white pith on the underside of the peel. Then, lay the peels in a basket or on a plate to dry. Once they're dry, store them in an airtight jar in a cool, dark place. If you live in a humid environment, you can bake the orange peels in a 150°F oven for 45 to 60 minutes to finish the drying process.

6. Rosemary stem–infused oil

Rosemary is a great herb to use in your skin- and hair-care routine. Rosemary has many benefits for the skin, including preventing acne, evening out skin tone, and reducing inflammation. Rosemary is also easy to find; you can grow it at home or buy it fresh at the grocery store. Rosemary oil is especially beneficial for hair and can help stimulate hair follicles and increase circulation to the scalp!

Method: Dry out rosemary stems and drop them inside your favorite plant oil. I love using apricot kernel oil for my skin, as it contains moisturizing and hydrating properties, but you can use avocado oil, grapeseed oil or any other light-weight plant oil.

PART II

Chapter 5
Customized Face Recipes

Our face helps us create that all-important first impression, but when we aren't proud of our face and skin—how it looks or feels—it affects our confidence in social settings. That's why I spend so much time helping people become better educated on how to take care of it.

Our face is greatly affected by air pollution, sun exposure, and the drying effects of heaters and air conditioners. The list of irritants that our faces come in contact with is endless. Facial skin suffers the most wear and tear on our entire body. It's easy to burden ourselves with a bunch of skin-care products for every organ of our face: eye cream, lip scrubs, facial serums, toners, mists, sheet masks, and the list goes on! In this digital age, we often blindly follow our favorite beauty bloggers to copy their daily rituals and recommendations of beauty products and implement them into our skin-care routines. But how can someone you've never met know what's best for your skin? They can't. After getting caught in this trap myself, I have hurt both my skin and my bank account—a lot.

The best and safest skin care starts in the kitchen. You already know from earlier chapters how to make the foundational, functional base formulas you'll see in the following pages. Using these base formulas, we will discuss how to turn everyday food scraps into precious and sustainable skin-care products. For example, you'll learn how to make an amazing facial mask using carrot tops, as they are packed with high chlorophyll, which can act as antioxidants and remove toxins from your skin. We'll make an eye mask from leftover eggshells for skin tightening near the eyes. And so much more!

Facial Cleansers

Facial cleansers are an important part of any skin-care routine. They help remove dirt, oil, and makeup from the skin, leaving it feeling refreshed and clean. Facial cleansers also help unclog pores and prevent breakouts. If you have sensitive skin, you want a facial cleanser that is gentle and nonirritating. For dry skin, you want a facial cleanser that is hydrating and contains ingredients like glycerin or hyaluronic acid. And for oily skin, you want a face wash that contains salicylic acid or other oil-absorbing ingredients. Having a cleansing ritual in the morning and at night using the following creams, balms, and oils is sure to improve your skin.

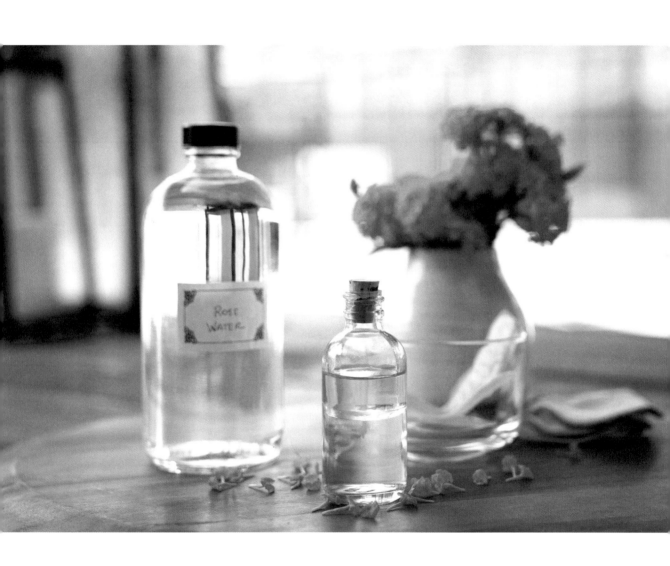

Bi-Phase Lemony Oil Cleanser

Shelf Life: Quantities are deliberately small to ensure that this product will be used within its shelf life. Keep it in the refrigerator for about 1 week. Similar commercial products contain preservatives, which is why they last longer, but this recipe focuses on freshness and health so its benefits will be longer-lasting.

A bi-phase makeup remover is a perfect way to start your cleansing routine. Using two phases, an oil phase and a water phase, this cleanser can effectively remove all traces of makeup, including waterproof formulas. Plus, it's gentle on the skin and won't leave your face feeling dry or stripped. Best of all, bi-phase makeup removers are typically made with natural, nontoxic ingredients that are good for you and the planet. So, if you're looking for a way to cleanse your face that is both effective and eco-friendly, a bi-phase makeup remover is the way to go.

Any cosmetic formula works with two phases: water and oil. To mix them more homogeneously, formulators typically use an emulsifier. To temporarily emulsify this cleaner, we'll simply shake the product for ten seconds to activate both phases. This process is safer, more sustainable, and more affordable.

The star ingredients of this recipe are Lemon Peel Glycerite and lemon peel–infused oil. While we generally throw away lemon peels, this part of the lemon contains vitamin C, citric acid, phytic acid, limonene, and certain enzymes, vitamins, and minerals. Lemon peel also contains antioxidants, which help combat free radicals, atoms in nature that can attack skin cells and damage the skin structure. Wrinkles, fine lines, and sagging result from free radical damage.

Ingredients

Phase	Amount	Role	Ingredients
Phase B	45% (0.45 ounce)	Foundational	Rose water
Phase B	5% (0.05 ounce)	Functional	Lemon Peel Glycerite (page 44)
Phase A	50% (.50 ounce)	Foundational	Lemon peel–infused oil (see Infusions on page 41)

(continued on next page)

Method

Mix rose water and Lemon Peel Glycerite in a small mixing jar with a lid. Once Phase B is mixed, add phase A (lemon peel–infused oil) on top of the water. Since the oil is heavy in molecules, it will float on top.

Superfood Green Cleanser

Shelf Life: Although this cleanser can last more than 1 month,
I suggest making a fresh one every month for best results.

This is a great pick-me-up for tired, lackluster skin. We use green tea bags in this recipe because green tea leaves are known for their antioxidant, anti-inflammatory, and antimicrobial properties. They help in fighting against premature aging, redness, and irritation and can treat acne, so this cleanser is great if you have oily, acne-prone, sun-damaged skin.

Ingredients

Phase	Amount	Role of Ingredient	Ingredients
Phase A	50% (50 ounces)	Foundational/functional	10 green tea bags
Phase A	25% (25 ounces)	Foundational/functional	Rice flour
Phase A	24% (24 ounces)	Functional	Ground almonds
Phase A	1% (1 ounce)	Aromatic	Rosemary essential oil

Method

Before you make anything using green tea, you must dehydrate the tea bags. I generally use a dehydrator to ensure the moisture is evaporated, but you can also dry the tea bags in the sun instead. Once dried, empty the contents and grind the tea leaves into a fine powder using a spice mixer. Now, mix the rice flour, ground almonds, and ground tea leaves. Finally, add the rosemary essential oil at the end. This cleanser has no lather, but it will clean your face like magic. Note: Don't get water in this cleanser (even with your wet fingers). It must stay dry until use. When you're ready to use it, simply activate the ingredients with water on your face.

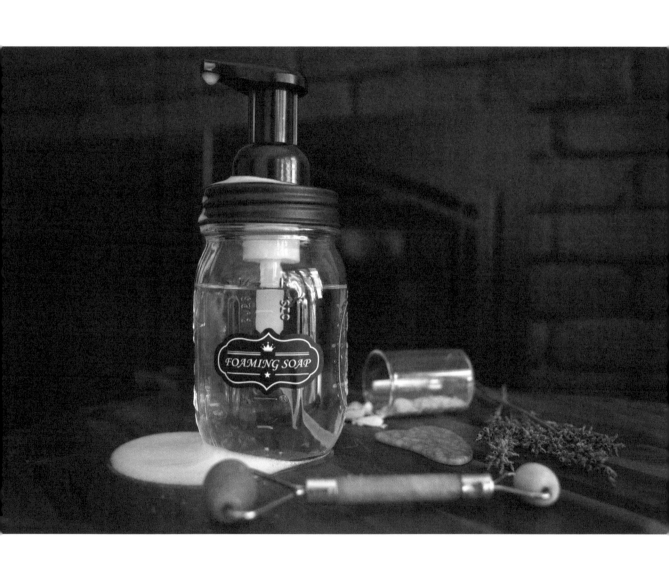

Foamy Exfoliating Cleanser

Shelf Life: This recipe has a shelf life of about 2 months. Castile soap contains natural preservatives, which will help keep this formula fresh for some time.

This recipe has no oil content and is beloved by those trying to avoid heavier oil-based cleansers. The secret to this recipe is in using a foam pump bottle. You can get a foam pump bottle online. The water base is filled with products inside the bottle, and the pump then pushes small amounts of product into the foam chamber, where the liquid and air mixture create a nice mousse/foam-like texture.

In conventional beauty products, surfactants (functional/botanical ingredients) are used to create a lather effect, but we will use simple castile soap (liquid soap made from natural ingredients such as coconut oil, hemp oil, and palm kernel oil) to achieve the same result in this recipe. As an exfoliator, we will use pistachio shell powder. Finally, we'll add in a few drops of lavender essential oil for great aroma and therapeutic value.

Ingredients

Phase	Amount	Role of Ingredient	Ingredients
Phase A	70% (70 ounces)	Foundational/functional	Castile soap
Phase A	19% (19 ounces)	Foundational/functional	Rose water
Phase A	10% (10 ounces)	Functional	Pistachio Shell Powder (page 45)
Phase A	1% (1 ounce)	Aromatic	Lavender essential oil

Method

Add castile soap and rose water into a foamer bottle and mix well. Then, mix in the pistachio shell powder. Finally, mix in the lavender essential oil.

Green Face Rinse

Shelf Life: This is a one-time application product. Use it immediately and discard the rest.

This face rinse comes from the extracted fibrous juice of kale stems blended with glycerin. Fun fact: The inspiration for this face rinse came when my mom insisted that I keep kale stems for our Indian chutney! Kale stems are rich in vitamins A, C, K, and E. This rinse is great to use when you want to rejuvenate your skin tone and reduce puffy eyes for the next morning. It promotes collagen production, increases cell generation, prevents free-radical damage, and detoxifies the skin.

Facial rinses, including this one, are generally water-based. The glycerin is added here to act as a humectant, which will lock the moisture into your face. This facial rinse is hydrating for dry skin types.

Ingredients

Phase	Amount	Role of Ingredient	Ingredients
Phase A	95% (90 ounces)	Foundational/functional	Kale stems
Phase A	5% (5 ounces)	Foundational	Filtered water
Phase B	5% (5 ounces)	Functional	Glycerin

Method

Blend the kale stems and filtered water in an immersion blender or food processor until you see a green liquid form. Filter the mixture using cheesecloth. Then, add in Phase B (glycerin) to the nice green liquid and mix well. To use this product, soak a cheesecloth in it and lay it over your face for 8 to 10 minutes, then rinse.

Orange Peel Cleansing Balm

Shelf Life: This cleansing balm will last approximately 3 months.
Make sure not to expose the product to any water.

Cleansing balm is popular because it acts as a cleanser and moisturizer all in one. Cleansing balms are perfect for dehydrated and dry skin. If you've ever felt itchy and dry after washing your face with conventional beauty products, this cleansing balm will be your savior! It works well because it rehydrates the skin.

The finished product will be thick, and once it comes into contact with water, it will create a beautiful, milky lather. Our magic ingredient is orange peel–infused almond oil. Orange peel is a popular ingredient in India, as it contains antioxidants. Regularly using it in a facial balm will give you clearer and brighter skin. This infused oil contains antibacterial and antimicrobial properties, making it great for treating acne-prone and oily skin. It's especially helpful to use if you live in colder or harsh climates.

Ingredients

Phase	Amount	Role of Ingredient	Ingredients
Phase A	5% (5 ounces)	Foundational	Emulsifying wax
Phase A	45% (45 ounces)	Foundational	Mango butter
Phase B	48% (48 ounces)	Foundational	Orange peel–infused almond oil (see Infusions on page 41)
Phase C	1% (1 ounce)	Additive	Vitamin E
Phase C	1% (1 ounce)	Aromatic	Sweet orange essential oil

Method

Gently melt the wax and mango butter in a double boiler or bain-marie. When melted, remove from heat and add in the orange peel–infused almond oil. Stir gently until the mixture reaches about room temperature or you see a trace on the edges of the pot. Next, add in the vitamin E and sweet orange essential oil. Keep stirring until the liquid is still runny but turning more

(continued on next page)

solid. Store in a wide-mouth jar with a lid. To use this product, place it directly around your eye area, forehead, neck, and jawline. Soak a cheesecloth in warm water and place the cloth on your face, pressing down gently for a few moments before cleansing and rinsing.

Carrot Peel Facial Cleanser

Shelf Life: This cleanser will keep for 3 months.

Vitamin C is one of the most vital tonics for removing dirt from your facial skin. Vitamin C is more concentrated in the carrot peels rather than in the carrot itself, which is why we're focusing on the peels in this recipe. This skin-care formula also contains castile soap because it is considered safe for even the most sensitive skin types and can help oily, acne-prone skin. (I recommend Dr. Bronner's Pure-Castile Soap. It's not a raw ingredient, but it's perfect for this recipe. Try to get the unscented one.) This recipe also consists of rosemary CO_2 extract or vitamin E and rosemary essential oil because they are excellent antioxidants and help remove all harmful substances from our skin!

Ingredients

Phase	Amount	Role of Ingredient	Ingredients
Phase A	85% (85 ounces)	Foundational	Castile soap
Phase A	13% (13 ounces)	Foundational	Carrot peel–infused rosehip oil (see Infusions on page 41)
Phase C	1% (1 ounce)	Additive	Rosemary CO_2 extract or vitamin E
Phase C	1% (1 ounce)	Aromatic	Rosemary essential oil

Method

Mix castile soap and carrot peel–infused rosehip oil in one container with a lid. Stir until it becomes homogeneous because the soap and oil need to be mixed properly. Then, add in rosemary CO_2 extract or vitamin E and rosemary essential oil. Shake it well. That's it! Your cleanser is ready.

You can customize this facial cleanser by using a different kind of oil. Instead of carrot peel–infused rosehip oil, use apple peel–infused oil, coriander–infused oil, or almond oil.

Moisturizers, Facial Oils, and Serums

One of the most important (and often underrated) products in your skin-care routine is facial moisturizer. A good facial moisturizer can do wonders for your skin, helping to keep it hydrated, plump, and smooth. It can also help protect your skin from environmental damage and reduce the appearance of fine lines and wrinkles. To keep your skin looking its best, you need to moisturize whether you have oily, sensitive, dry, or combination skin.

In this section, you will learn how to make different moisturizers. For the most potent, I'll give you the recipe for an easy water-free moisturizer. I will also introduce a few facial oils and serums for your AM and PM rituals. Facial oil is a mixture of botanical oils, macerated oils, oil-soluble extracts, and essential oils. I generally use facial oils for nighttime nourishment, as they have thick molecules that soak into your skin throughout the night. Serums are similar to facial oils, but they contain more concentrated ingredients and finer oils.

Anhydrous Minty Moisturizer

Shelf Life: This moisturizer will keep for up to 3 months. Keep away from all heat.

Like most people, you've probably struggled with acne at some point in your life. Acne is the most common skin problem in the United States, affecting millions of Americans annually. While there are many possible causes of acne, the most common culprit is the overproduction of oil. This excess oil can clog pores and provide a perfect breeding ground for bacteria. Other factors contributing to acne include hormonal imbalances, stress, and certain medications. Fortunately, there are many effective treatments for those who suffer from acne. Green beauty products and sustainable beauty practices are becoming increasingly popular among people looking for natural solutions to their skin problems.

This moisturizer is perfect for acne-prone skin because it contains all the goodies that can resolve acne. Mint stems are great for addressing acne scars and cleaning the pores. The comedogenic score of grapeseed oil is 1, which means it won't clog your pores and will help improve the skin barrier.

Ingredients

Phase	Amount	Role of Ingredient	Ingredients
Phase A	50% (50 ounces)	Foundational	Mint stem–infused grapeseed oil (see Infusions on page 41)
Phase A	49% (48 ounces)	Foundational	Shea butter
Phase B	1% (1 ounce)	Additive	Vitamin E
Phase B	1% (1 ounce)	Aromatic	Tea tree essential oil

Method

Gently melt mint stem–infused grapeseed oil and shea butter in a double boiler or bain-marie. Remove from heat and let cool, then put into the freezer for 2 to 5 minutes. Once trace forms, blend the mixture with an immersion blender or hand blender. Then, add in vitamin E and tea tree essential oil and stir until mixture hardens. Put it into the freezer for another couple of minutes if you think your cream is on the runny side. Transfer it to a jar with a lid and label with the date.

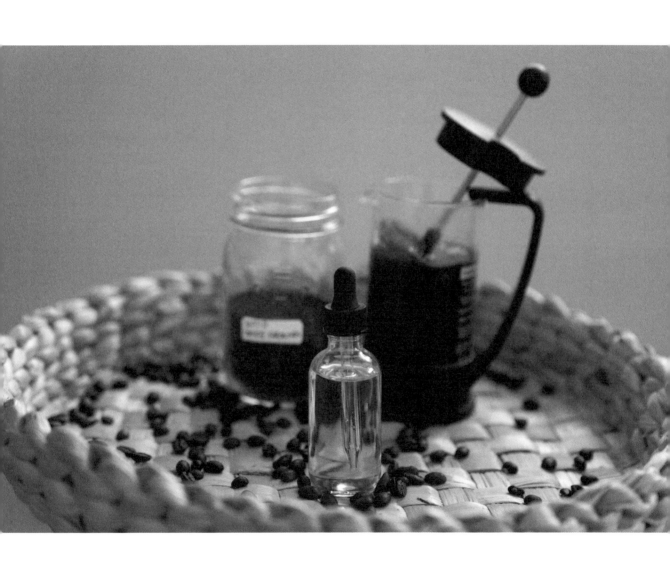

Wrinkle-Free Oil Serum

Shelf Life: This oil serum will keep for 1 month. Keep it away from heat.

The antioxidants and caffeine found in coffee grounds can help reduce the appearance of wrinkles, improve blood circulation, and reduce inflammation. When applied topically, coffee grounds can also tighten and tone the skin. So next time you brew a pot of coffee, don't throw out the grounds—put them to good use and give your skin a little extra boost! This highly effective oil serum helps reduce the appearance of puffy eyes. The great thing about this recipe is that it contains just three simple ingredients.

Ingredients

Phase	Amount	Role of Ingredient	Ingredients
Phase A	98% (98 ounces)	Foundational	Used coffee ground–infused argan oil (see Infusions on page 41)
Phase B	1% (1 ounce)	Additive	Vitamin E
Phase B	1% (1 ounce)	Aromatic	Tea tree essential oil

Method

Mix used coffee ground–infused argan oil, vitamin E, and tea tree essential oil together. Store this product in a wide-mouth jar with a lid. To use this product, massage thoroughly and gently for 1 minute after applying toner and cleanser. Repeat daily.

Oil-Free Facial Lotion Spray

Shelf Life: Keep this lotion refrigerated for up to 1 month.

If you have acne-prone skin, you know the importance of using oil-free products. Oil-free lotions are often lighter and less greasy than traditional lotions, making them a good choice for people who don't like the feel of heavy products on their skin. Ultimately, oil-free lotions are a great option for anyone who wants to keep their skin healthy and acne-free.

Spray this lotion onto your face and neck and get a shiny golden and pinkish glow on your skin. This facial lotion has no oil, but the beetroot scrap glycerite will give your skin a shiny glow.

Ingredients

Phase	Amount	Role of Ingredient	Ingredients
Phase A	54% (54 ounces)	Foundational	Rose water
Phase A	45% (45 ounces)	Functional/foundational	Beetroot scrap glycerite (see Glycerites on page 42)
Phase B	1% (1 ounce)	Extra	Vitamin E

Method

Combine rose water and beetroot scrap glycerite together in a spray bottle. Then, add vitamin E. Gently shake the bottle or use a glass rod to blend everything together.

Herby Facial Oil

Shelf Life: Keep this oil no more than 3 months.

People often wonder if they should apply facial oil before or after their moisturizer. With this herby facial oil, you can forget about moisturizers altogether! This recipe uses coriander, parsley, and mint stems. Coriander stems contain skin-boosting vitamin C, complexion-friendly minerals, and many other botanical benefits. Mint stems are a potent source of antibacterial, antiseptic, and antifungal disinfectants. The parsley stems in this herbal oil act as a natural skin enhancer since it contains a high amount of vitamin C.

Ingredients

Phase	Amount	Role of Ingredient	Ingredients
Phase A	33% (33 ounces)	Functional/foundational	Coriander stem–infused almond oil (see Infusions on page 41)
Phase A	33% (33 ounces)	Functional/foundational	Mint stem–infused sunflower oil (see Infusions on page 41)
Phase A	31% (31 ounces)	Functional/foundational	Parsley stem–infused sunflower oil (see Infusions on page 41)
Phase B	1% (1 ounce)	Additive	Vitamin E
Phase B	1% (1 ounce)	Aromatic	Lemongrass essential oil

Method

Mix the infused oils together. Then, add in vitamin E and lemongrass essential oil. Pour the mixture in a dropper bottle and shake. You'll need only two drops for your face and neck. This oil should be applied on clean skin by gently pressing your fingers on the face to absorb all the botanical benefits into skin. You can also add this oil to your regular moisturizer for extra hydration.

Fruity Facial Oil

Shelf Life: This oil will last for 3 months.

Muggy summers can lead to closed pores and breakouts, so a good after-sun facial oil is essential during this time of year. This facial oil aims to provide relief after a day in the sun and protect against sun damage and premature aging. Fruit peels contain vitamin C (an antiaging superstar), niacinamide (vitamin B3), and citric acid (in the family of alpha-hydroxy acids).

Ingredients

Phase	Amount	Role of Ingredient	Ingredients
Phase A	45% (45 ounces)	Functional/foundational	Fruit peel–infused almond oil (see Infusions on page 41)
Phase A	45% (40 ounces)	Functional/foundational	Fractionated coconut oil
Phase A	5% (10 ounces)	Functional/foundational	Castor oil
Phase B	2% (1 ounce)	Additive	Vitamin E
Phase B	1% (1 ounce)	Aromatic	Sweet orange essential oil
Phase B	1% (1 ounce)	Aromatic	Bergamot essential oil

Method

First, combine all Phase A ingredients in one beaker. In another beaker, combine all Phase B ingredients. Then, combine Phases A and B together and pour them into an airless pump bottle or a simple dropper bottle. Add this oil to your regular moisturizer for extra hydration.

Other Facial Recipes

If you are looking for an easy, affordable, and transparent way to upgrade your beauty routine, the following at-home facial recipes are the answer. Whether it's an indulgent lip scrub or eye mask, these simple yet powerful recipes can be whipped up right in the comfort of your home.

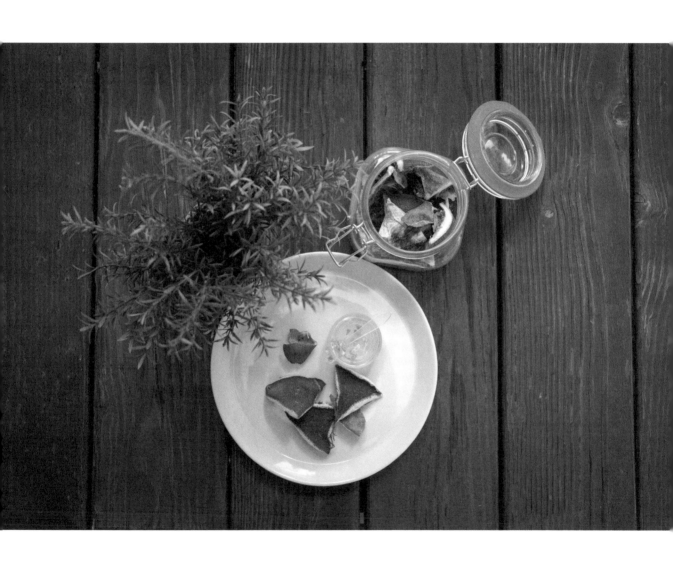

Dark Circle–Removing Eye Gel

Shelf Life: Keep this product in the refrigerator for up to 15 days.

We all know that getting a good night's sleep is important for our overall health, but did you know that it can also help improve the appearance of your skin? One benefit of a good night's sleep is that it can help reduce the appearance of dark circles under your eyes. When we're tired, our skin looks paler and more translucent, which allows the blood vessels beneath the skin to show through. This can give the skin a bruised or sunken appearance. Getting enough sleep helps to improve circulation and gives the skin a chance to repair itself, which can help reduce the appearance of dark circles.

If you're looking to brighten up your complexion, the best way is to get plenty of rest, but this dark circle–removing eye gel offers a quick and easy fix. The star ingredient in this recipe is orange peel, which acts as an antioxidant and skin-brightening agent. Orange peel glycerite will allow this eye gel to absorb right into your skin, making it ideal to use before putting on your makeup for the day. It's excellent for calming morning puffiness and reducing dark circles, as it energizes and refreshes the skin.

Ingredients

Phase	Amount	Role of Ingredient	Ingredients
Phase A	5% (5 ounces)	Functional/foundational	Agar agar (find this product online or at your local grocery store)
Phase A	45% (55 ounces)	Functional/foundational	Orange peel glycerite (see Glycerites on page 42)
Phase A	45% (40 ounces)	Functional/foundational	Distilled or filtered water

Method

In a bowl, combine the agar agar with the glycerite. Slowly add in the distilled or filtered water and mix until the consistency is gel-like. I suggest using this eye gel on a weekly basis.

Potato Peel Eye Slushies

Shelf Life: This recipe is for one-time use.

Potato peels contain properties that give off a cooling effect and reduce inflammation near the eyes so, instead of throwing away your potato peels, make super calming eye slushies out of them!

Ingredients

Phase	Amount	Role of Ingredient	Ingredients
Phase A	45% (10 ounces)	Functional/foundational	Potato peels, washed
Phase A	80% (90 ounces)	Functional/foundational	Distilled or filtered water

Method

Arrange the potato peels in an ice cube tray, fill with distilled or filtered water, and stick in the freezer. Once they become potato peel ice cubes, put two cubes into a cloth, and muddle with a muddler until ice is crushed. Wrap slushie in the cloth and rest over your eyes.

Sweet Rosy Face Detox

Shelf Life: This is a one-time only mask. Both sets of ingredients will keep in the refrigerator for 2 months.

Sweet potatoes are an unusually nutritional vegetable, a rich source of vitamins A, C, E, and K. I love using sweet potato as a beauty ingredient because the peels help neutralize free radicals that cause oxidative stress. They contain vitamin A, a natural form of retinol that reduces fine lines, wrinkles, blemishes, sagging skin, and the list goes on. Rose petal powder works to minimize uneven skin tone and brighten the skin. Aloe vera gel acts as a humectant, and rose water is the activating ingredient.

Ingredients

Phase	Amount	Role of Ingredient	Ingredients
Phase A	60% (60 ounces)	Functional	Sweet Potato Peel Powder (page 44)
Phase A	40% (40 ounces)	Functional	Rose petal powder

Phase	Amount	Role of Ingredient	Ingredients
Phase B	90% (90 ounces)	Functional	Rose water
Phase B	10% (10 ounces)	Functional	Aloe vera gel

Method

Mix Phase A ingredients together in a jar with a lid. In a separate jar with a lid, mix Phase B ingredients together. To use this product, weigh 10 ounces of the powdered ingredients in a glass bowl, then add 10 milliliters of the liquid ingredients to activate. Blend well until smooth and easy to spread. Add more liquid if needed. Apply this mask to your clean face and leave on for 10 minutes. It's perfect for when you want an instant glow and to reduce all the fine lines.

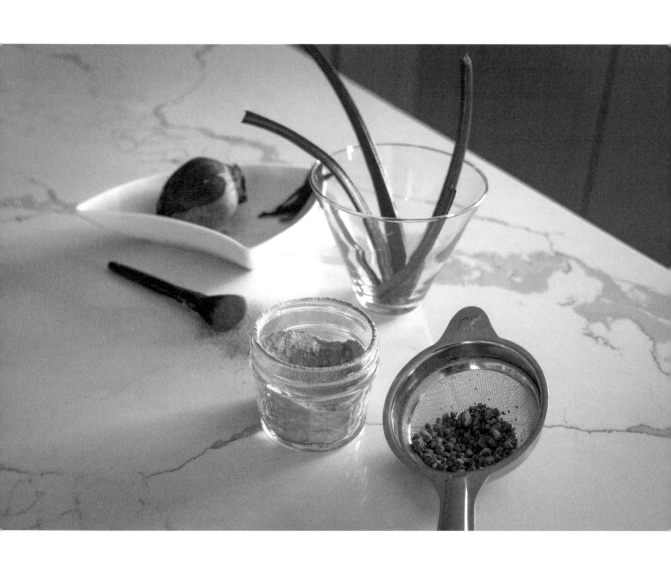

Beetroot Blush

Shelf Life: This blush will last approximately 3 to 4 months.

While the zero-waste movement has been gaining momentum in recent years, many products are still difficult to find in zero-waste form. One of the most challenging categories is makeup. Many conventional makeup products are packaged in single-use plastic containers, and even those that come in recyclable packaging often contain a mix of materials that makes them difficult to recycle. We'll use nontoxic, harmless ingredients in this recipe to make your cheeks rosy and blush. You can also use this product to add highlights to your hair.

Ingredients

Phase	Amount	Role of Ingredient	Ingredients
Phase A	40% (40 ounces)	Foundational	Rice flour
Phase A	18% (18 ounces)	Functional/foundational	Arrowroot powder
Phase A	40% (40 ounces)	Functional/foundational	Beetroot powder
Phase B	2% (2 ounces)	Additive	Pink eye shadow, crushed (optional)

Method

Using a sifter, sift the rice and arrowroot powders. Mix them well to separate the lumps. Then, sift the beetroot powder and mix again. To give this blush a little shine, add a touch of pink eye shadow.

Fruit Scraps Facial Steam

Shelf Life: Generally, steams should be used immediately, but the strained water can also be stored in the fridge for 1 to 2 weeks.

Save all your citrus fruit scraps for this practical and sustainable face steam. This is a fantastic recipe to deep-pore cleanse and detoxify your skin. The bioflavonoids from the fruit peels are excellent preventative remedies for skin.

Ingredients

Phase	Amount	Role of Ingredient	Ingredients
Phase A	92% (92 ounces)	Foundational	Distilled water
Phase A	2% (2 ounces)	Functional	Lime peels
Phase A	2% (2 ounces)	Functional	Lemon peels
Phase A	2% (2 ounces)	Functional	Orange peels
Phase A	2% (2 ounces)	Functional	Grapefruit peels

Method

In a small pan, heat the water until simmering. Add all the fruit peels into the facial steam and let simmer for 4 to 5 minutes. Strain the water into a large bowl and allow it to cool for 1 to 2 minutes, or enough to avoid accidental burns. Place a towel over your head and lower your face until you are about 8 to 12 inches from the bowl. Keep your head far enough away from the steam so that it is a warm mist, never hot, and steam for 5 minutes. After your steam, dab your face with a clean cloth.

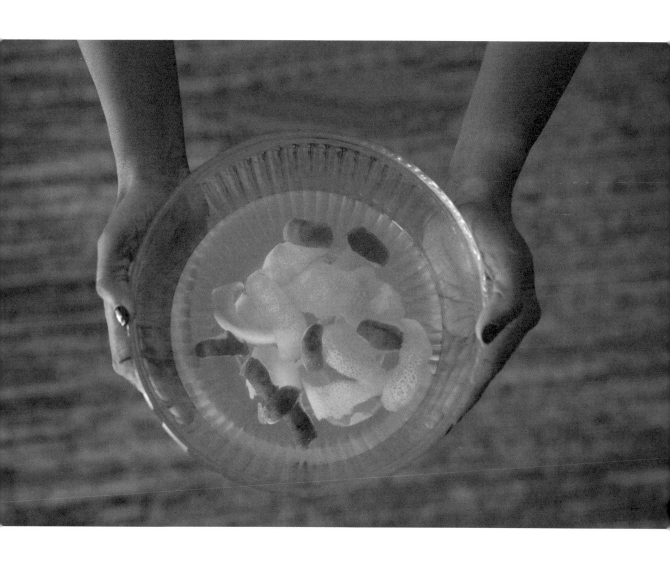

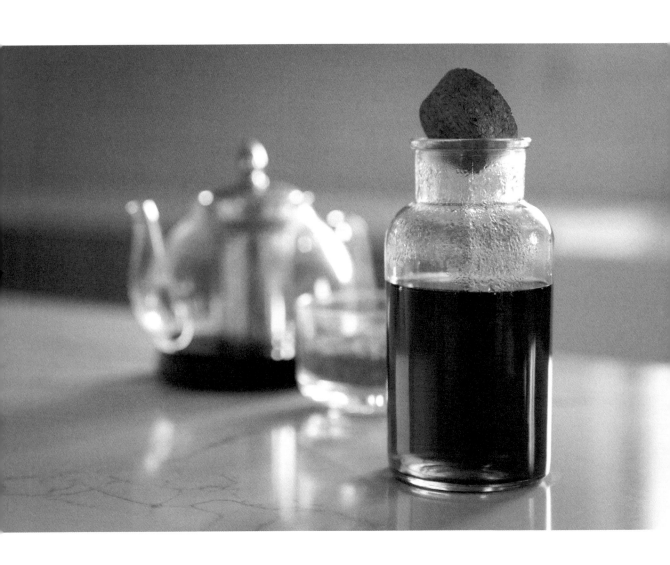

Red Lentil Toner

Shelf Life: This toner will last up to 1 week and must be refrigerated.

Toner can balance out the skin's pH after using alkaline-heavy products like bar soap or cleansing soap. Store-bought toners are generally water or alcohol-based, but in this recipe, we use leftover red lentil water to make an amazing facial toner. Red lentils provide a brightening effect on your skin.

Ingredients

Phase	Amount	Role of Ingredient	Ingredients
Phase A	60% (60 ounces)	Functional	Red lentil water
Phase A	35% (35 ounces)	Functional/foundational	Red raspberry tea, cold and brewed
Phase A	3% (3 ounces)	Functional	Aloe vera gel
Phase B	2% (2 ounces)	Aromatic	Rose essential oil

Method

Mix the red lentil water with red raspberry tea, then add in aloe vera gel and blend well. Finally, add your rose essential oil and mix. Pour into a spray bottle. When you want to use this toner, mix it well and spray it all over your face. It's best used right after you cleanse your face or after using a mask or facial scrub. It will open your pores and prepare you for the next step in your skin-care ritual (i.e., moisturizer).

Cucumber Peel Facial Mist

Shelf Life: This facial mist will last up to 1 week and must be refrigerated.

This toner is a great addition to your summertime skin-care routine because the high-water content in cucumber peels helps to keep the skin hydrated and nourished. The skin benefits of cucumber peels are plentiful. They contain antioxidants, enzymes, and minerals like potassium, magnesium, and silicon that help improve skin complexion and reduce wrinkles.

Ingredients

Phase	Amount	Role of Ingredient	Ingredients
Phase A	80% (80 ounces)	Functional/foundational	Rose water/your favorite hydrosol
Phase A	18% (18 ounces)	Functional/foundational	Cucumber peel glycerite (see Glycerites on page 42)
Phase A	2% (2 ounces)	Functional/foundational	Vitamin E

Method

Measure rose water or your favorite hydrosol into a spray bottle. Using a funnel, slowly add in the cucumber peel glycerite and vitamin E. When you want to use this toner, mix it well and spray it all over your face. It's best used right after you cleanse your face or after using a mask or facial scrub. It will open your pores and prepare you for the next step in your skin-care ritual (i.e., moisturizer).

Mango Seed Face Mask

Shelf Life: This is a one-time only mask. Both sets of ingredients will keep in the refrigerator for 2 months.

Growing up in India, mango was always the most loved fruit at our house! Since you can't get this fruit year-round in India, we always had to wait until summer, but I always kept mango seed powder on hand for all my beauty needs. After you eat the mango, the leftover seeds can be dried in the sunlight. Once it's dry, the powder of the seed is a great ingredient for skincare. Mango seed powder has powerful antimicrobial properties. It clears your skin from stubborn acne and pimples that can cause embarrassment. Kaolin clay is great for removing excess oil from the skin, and strawberry powder provides a brightening and cooling effect.

Ingredients

Phase	Amount	Role of Ingredient	Ingredients
Phase A	40% (40 ounces)	Functional	Kaolin clay
Phase A	30% (30 ounces)	Functional	Mango seed powder (see Powdered Herbal Scraps on page 37)
Phase A	30% (30 ounces)	Functional	Strawberry powder (see Powdered Herbal Scraps on page 37)

Phase	Amount	Role of Ingredient	Ingredients
Phase B	90% (90 ounces)	Foundational	Distilled water
Phase B	10% (10 ounces)	Functional	Vegetable glycerite (see Glycerites on page 42)

Method

Mix all Phase A ingredients in a jar with a lid. In a separate jar with a lid, mix all Phase B ingredients. To use this product, weigh 10 ounces of the powdered ingredients in a glass bowl, then add 10 milliliters of the liquid ingredients to activate. Blend well until smooth and easy to spread. Add more liquid if needed. Apply this mask to your clean face and leave on for 10 minutes.

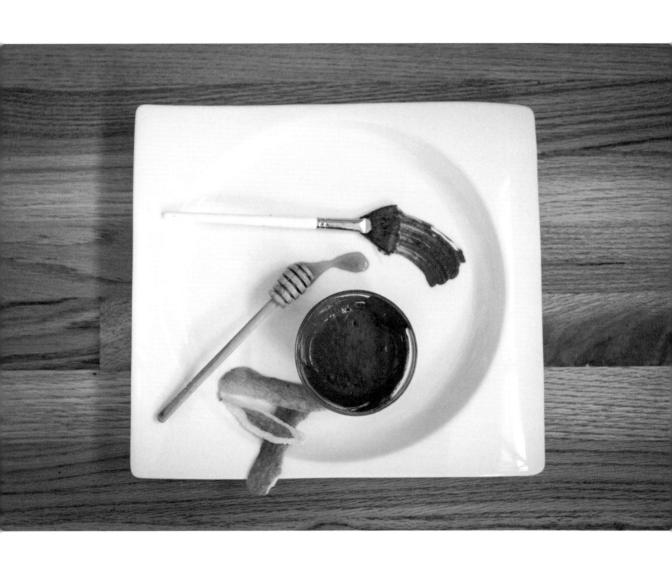

Revitalizing Face Mask

Shelf Life: This is a one-time only mask. Both sets of ingredients will keep in the refrigerator for 2 months.

Next time you're looking for a beauty boost, don't reach for synthetic products—head to your kitchen instead! There are plenty of zero-waste, sustainable options waiting for you. My favorite is pomegranate for its beautiful color and skin and health benefits. Pomegranate is high in antioxidants, which protect your skin from free radicals and environmental pollution and reduce wrinkles and age spots. Pomegranate peels are also high in vitamin C, which helps keep your skin healthy and youthful looking. If you live in cities or an urbanized area, save every single leftover you have from this fruit.

Ingredients

Phase	Amount	Role of Ingredient	Ingredients
Phase A	40% (40 ounces)	Functional	Fuller's earth
Phase A	30% (30 ounces)	Functional	Pomegranate peel powder (see Powdered Herbal Scraps on page 37)
Phase A	30% (30 ounces)	Functional	Coconut milk powder

Phase	Amount	Role of Ingredient	Ingredients
Phase B	90% (90 ounces)	Foundational	Rose water
Phase B	10% (10 ounces)	Functional	Honey

Method

Mix all Phase A ingredients together in a jar with a lid. In a separate jar with a lid, mix all Phase B ingredients together. To use this product, weigh 10 ounces of the powdered ingredients in a glass bowl, then add 10 milliliters of the liquid ingredients to activate. Blend well until smooth and easy to spread. Add more liquid if needed. Apply this mask to your clean face and leave on for 10 to 12 minutes. Remove this mask with a warm, wet napkin to give you a double-down effect of facial steam and face mask.

Grapefruit Peel Lip Scrub

Shelf Life: This is a one-time only scrub.
Store the powdered ingredients separately in a dark place up to 1 month.

I start my day by using a lip scrub to exfoliate my lips and then follow with a lip balm. This routine has helped my lips stay hydrated and soft. I also use a lip scrub before applying lipstick or lip gloss to ensure that my lips are smooth and free of dry skin.

Compared to the rest of your face, the skin on your lips is the most fragile, delicate, and sensitive. This lip scrub recipe is made with just a few simple ingredients, and because we are dealing with the mouth area, all ingredients are edible.

Ingredients

Phase	Amount	Role of Ingredient	Ingredients
Phase A	60% (60 ounces)	Functional	Coconut oil
Phase A	40% (40 ounces)	Functional	Grapefruit peel powder (see Powdered Herbal Scraps on page 37)

Method

Simply mix coconut oil and grapefruit peel powder together. To use, remove any lip color, lipstick, or lip balm first. Wash your lips with warm water, then apply this scrub in a circular motion for 2 minutes. Wash and apply lip balm immediately after.

Facial Detox

Facial detox is all about using green, sustainable, and natural products to cleanse and nourish your skin. It's about taking a holistic approach to beauty and wellness, and it starts with the basic premise that what you put on your skin should be good enough to eat. Your skin is your largest organ, and everything you put on it is absorbed into your body. So why not give it the nourishment it needs to function at its best?

When you detox your face, you're not only giving your skin the nutrients it needs to thrive; you're also giving yourself a chance to relax and unplug from the constant onslaught of messages telling you that you're not good enough as you are. A facial detox is an act of self-care, and it's one we all deserve to experience.

This mask is my favorite way to detox! It's made up of a simple blend of botanical ingredients to make you glow. Kaolin clay is one of the most versatile cosmetic clays, as it absorbs all impurities. Yogurt contains vitamin E, lactic acid, and beta-hydroxy acids. Spinach stems are rich in vitamins A, B6, C, calcium, iron, and magnesium and are great at protecting your skin from UV rays, enhancing your skin's complexion, and delaying signs of ageing.

Ingredients

Phase	Amount	Role of Ingredient	Ingredients
Phase A	70% (70 ounces)	Functional	Kaolin clay
Phase A	30% (30 ounces)	Functional	Spinach stem powder (see Powdered Herbal Scraps on page 37)

Phase	Amount	Role of Ingredient	Ingredients
Phase B	100% (90 ounces)	Foundational	Yogurt

(continued on next page)

Method

Mix both Phase A ingredients together in a wide-mouth jar with a lid. For Phase B, I prefer to use it fresh or as needed. To use this product, weigh 10 ounces of the powdered ingredients in a glass bowl, then add in 10 milliliters of the liquid ingredient. Blend well until smooth and easy to spread. The goal here is to use both phases fifty-fifty. Apply this mask to your clean face and leave on for 10 minutes.

Probiotic Face Scrub

Shelf Life: Made to use.

This is my rescue mask when my skin feels dull and I want immediate results! In this recipe, Greek yogurt takes center stage.

Ingredients

Phase	Amount	Role of Ingredient	Ingredients
Phase A	50% (50 ounces)	Functional	Greek yogurt
Phase A	30% (30 ounces)	Functional	Grapefruit peel powder (see Powdered Herbal Scraps on page 37)
Phase A	20% (20 ounces)	Functional	Bentonite clay powder

Method

This face mask is as simple as it looks. Just take a small mixing bowl and mix all ingredients together. Apply this face mask once a week to get gentle exfoliation from the lactic acid found inside Greek yogurt.

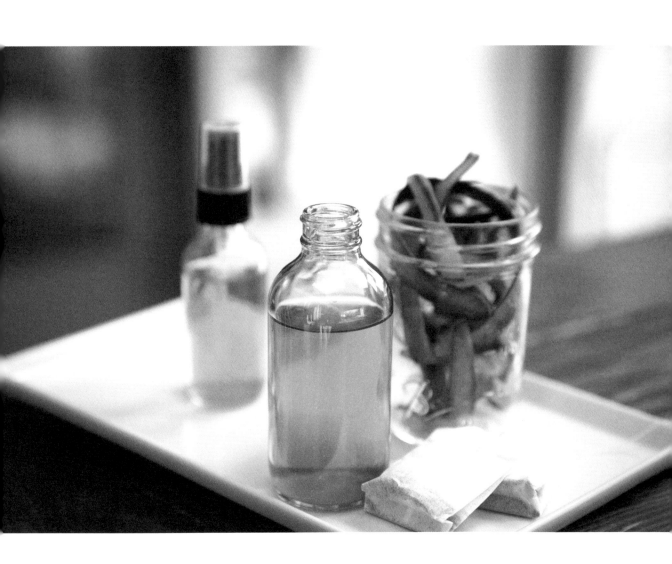

Cucumber and Mint Toner

Shelf Life: This toner will last for 1 week and must be refrigerated.

Cucumber and mint are a killer combo in my kitchen. It immediately gives me a refreshing feeling, whether in drinks or in this toner. This recipe is inspired by those hot summer days, and it's very easy to whip up once you have your ingredients ready to go.

Ingredients

Phase	Amount	Role of Ingredient	Ingredients
Phase A	60% (60 ounces)	Functional	Boiled water
Phase A	35% (35 ounces)	Functional/foundational	Green tea, brewed and chilled
Phase A	3% (3 ounces)	Functional	Cucumber glycerite (see Glycerites on page 42)
Phase B	2% (2 ounces)	Aromatic	Spearmint essential oil

Method

Mix boiled water with green tea, then add in cucumber glycerite and blend really well. Finally, add in spearmint essential oil and mix. Add this mixture to a spray bottle. To use, mix really well and spray all over your face. This toner is best used right after you cleanse your face or after using a mask or facial scrub. It will open your pores and make you ready for the next step in your skin-care ritual (i.e., moisturizer).

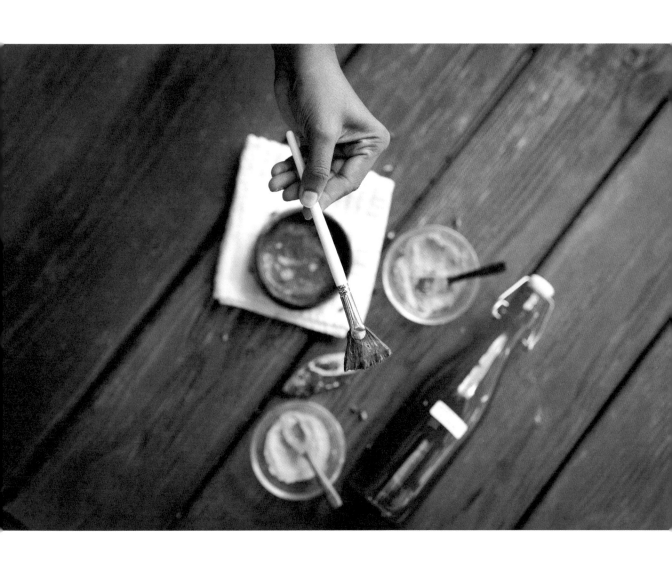

Brightening Face Mask

Shelf Life: Made to use.

Vinegar, clay, and herbal scraps: This trio acts as magic for every type of skin.

Ingredients

Phase	Amount	Role of Ingredient	Ingredients
Phase A	50% (50 ounces)	Functional	Bentonite clay
Phase A	30% (30 ounces)	Functional	Pomegranate peel powder (see Powdered Herbal Scraps on page 37)
Phase A	20% (20 ounces)	Functional	Apple cider vinegar

Method

Add bentonite clay, pomegranate peel powdcr, and apple cider vinegar to a small mixing bowl. Then, slowly add water to create a thick paste-like face mask. Apply this face mask once a week.

Chapter 6
Bath and Body Recipes

One of the simplest and most effective forms of self-care is taking care of our bodies. This includes everything from eating healthy foods and exercising regularly to getting enough sleep and managing stress. Although these activities may seem mundane, they play an important role in keeping us physically and mentally healthy. By taking care of our bodies, we also take care of our skin—the largest organ in our bodies. When we nourish our skin with healthy ingredients and provide it with adequate hydration, we are not only improving our appearance but also supporting our overall health. This chapter includes DIY bath and body recipes to help you in your quest for sustainably clean and radiant skin.

Body Cleansers

Body cleansers not only help you stay clean and provide a pleasant aroma but can also impact your overall skin health. A good cleanse will remove dirt, sweat, and other contaminants from your skin. From locked-in moisture to nourishing ingredients that protect against bacteria and dirt, the following recipes offer advantages over their store-bought competitors!

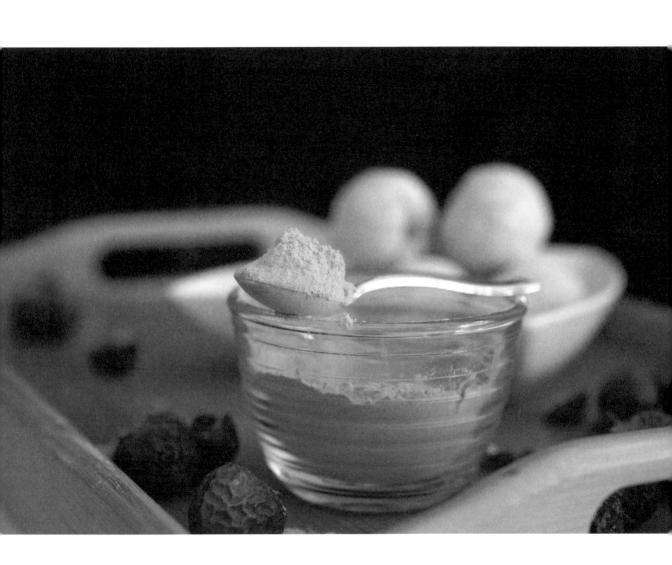

Dry Ayurvedic Soap Powder

Shelf Life: This powder will last about 1 month. Make sure it does not come into contact with water before use.

Ayurvedic soaps differ from other soaps, as they keep the skin healthy and fresh without harmful substances. This dry ayurvedic soap powder is good for the body because it has natural antibacterial agents that are useful in keeping germs away from the skin and preventing skin problems like acne and early aging.

Ingredients

Phase	Amount	Role of Ingredient	Ingredients
Phase A	5% (5 ounces)	Foundational	Soapnut powder
Phase A	45% (45 ounces)	Foundational	Oatmeal, ground
Phase B	48% (48 ounces)	Functional/utilitarian	Pomegranate peel powder (see Powdered Herbal Scraps on page 37)
Phase C	1% (1 ounce)	Additive	Vitamin E
Phase C	1% (1 ounce)	Aromatic	Lemon essential oil

Method

This recipe calls for a good coffee grinder. Add soapnut powder, oats, and pomegranate peel powder to the coffee grinder and grind until very fine. Then, add in vitamin E and lemon essential oil and grind once more. When done grinding, wait ten minutes before opening the coffee grinder.

Probiotic Citrusy Gel Soap

Shelf Life: This soap will last for about 1 month.
Make sure it does not come into contact with water before use.

Probiotic soap serves as an immune system for the skin. This probiotic citrusy gel soap is rich in vitamin E, making it effective in reducing the effects of aging because of sunlight; preventing and treating skin problems like eczema, acne, and atopic dermatitis; and taking care of allergic reactions and wounds on the skin. It has a mild effect on the skin and does not remove the important microbiome that protects it. It works for all parts of the body, and also comes with a sweet-smelling scent.

Ingredients

Phase	Amount	Role of Ingredient	Ingredients
Phase A	70% (70 ounces)	Foundational	Unscented castile soap
Phase A	10% (10 ounces)	Foundational	Grapefruit peel powder (see Powdered Herbal Scraps on page 37)
Phase B	7% (7 ounces)	Functional/utilitarian	Agar jelly or agar agar powder
Phase C	2% (2 ounces)	Additive	Probiotic capsule powder
Phase C	1% (1 ounce)	Aromatic	Orange or lemon essential oil

Method

Measure unscented castile soap in a small jar or container. Add grapefruit peel powder and agar jelly or agar agar. Mix well and let sit for 10 to 15 minutes until mixture is thick. Then, add probiotic capsule powder and essential oil of choice. To use this soap in the shower, apply to the body and leave it to dry for about 1 to 2 minutes before rinsing off. Then, use a cleansing cloth or loofah to exfoliate your skin gently. To use in the bathtub, put the desired quantity of gel into the bathtub before getting in.

Easy Peasy Coffee Lotion Bar for All Skin Types

Shelf Life: This coffee lotion bar will last 10 to 12 months.

Lotions bars are a great zero-waste choice for sustainable beauty, and you can make them in a wide variety of fun and invigorating scents. They're easy to transport, and because they're package-free, you can feel good about using them without contributing to plastic pollution.

This formula is a combination of ground coffee, which helps to reduce inflammation on the skin like eczema and acne, with cocoa butter rich in fatty acids, which moisturize the skin. It is mixed with shea butter that makes the skin soft while treating skin conditions like rashes, eczema, and irritation, among others.

Ingredients

Phase	Amount	Role of Ingredient	Ingredients
Phase A	70% (44 ounces)	Foundational	Cocoa butter
Phase A	20% (54 ounces)	Functional/utilitarian	Shea butter
Phase A	8% (1 ounce)	Functional/utilitarian	Used coffee ground–infused jojoba oil (see Infusions on page 41)
Phase B	2% (1 ounce)	Antioxidant	Vitamin E

Method

Melt the butters in a double boiler or bain-marie. When molten, remove from heat and let cool slightly, then add in the oil and vitamin E. Continue stirring until the mixture begins to solidify but is still pourable. Pour the mixture into soap molds or muffin molds and leave to set for at least 12 to 15 hours. Once solid, remove the bars from the molds and wrap them in parchment paper.

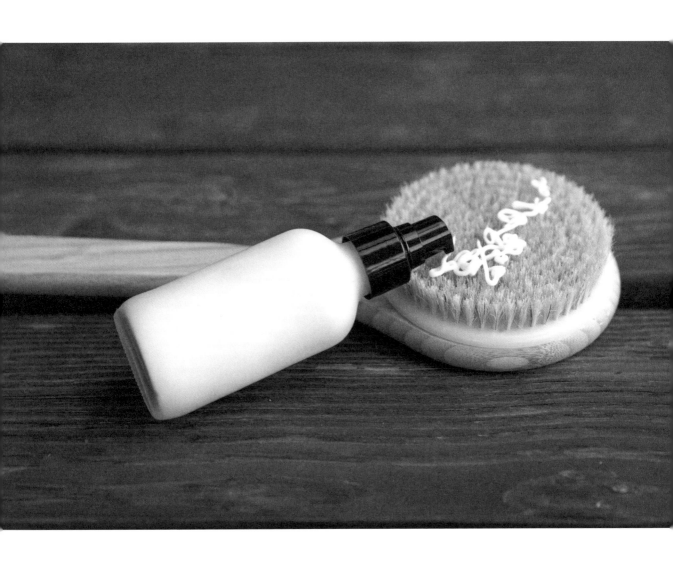

Creamy Liquid Soap

Shelf Life: This soap will last from to 1 to 3 months.

If you have dry skin, this formula is for you. Its mild texture does not dry out on the skin, and it also removes eczema, acne, body irritation, and rashes from the body. Its aloe vera content also repairs rough skin that could have been caused by wind or cold weather exposure. With this product, you will get the skin texture and glow you have always wanted.

Ingredients

Phase	Amount	Role of Ingredient	Ingredients
Phase A	5% (5 ounces)	Foundational	Grapeseed or any lightweight carrier oil
Phase A	70% (70 ounces)	Foundational	Aloe vera gel
Phase B	20% (20 ounces)	Functional/utilitarian	Unscented castile soap
Phase C	3% (3 ounces)	Additive	Epsom salt or table salt
Phase C	2% (2 ounces)	Additive	Vitamin E

Method

In a small bowl, mix the oil and aloe vera gel. Whisk it fast to develop a nice cream-based consistency. In a separate bowl, add the castile soap and salt and whisk until the soap becomes thicker. Combine the soap and aloe vera gel mixtures to make it a nice milky soap. Add in vitamin E.

Coconut Oat Exfoliating Soap

Shelf Life: This soap will last for 3 to 6 months.

To free your skin of dirt, oils, debris, redness, irritation, and dryness, this soap is a no-brainer and is one of my favorites, as it is rich in anti-inflammatory, antibacterial, and antifungal properties. Oatmeal, an ingredient with an abundance of protein, saponin, and lipids, enables this soap to work as an efficient skin cleanser that is smooth and soft on the body. It does not end there; oatmeal's antipruritic properties deal with inflammatory problems on the skin. Paired with the properties of banana peel, rich in vitamin C and antioxidants, this soap helps boost your skin's elasticity to give you clean and glowing skin.

Ingredients

Phase	Amount	Role of Ingredient	Ingredients
Phase A	82% (82 ounces)	Foundational	Any vegan melt-and-pour soap base (coconut is my favorite)
Phase A	13% (13 ounces)	Functional	Banana peel powder (see Powdered Herbal Scraps on page 37)
Phase B	2% (2 ounces)	Additive	French pink clay
Phase B	2% (2 ounces)	Functional/ utilitarian	Any lightweight carrier oil infused with any citrus peel
Phase B	1% (1 ounce)	Aromatic	Lemon essential oil

Method

Cut your soap base into small pieces and add them to a heatproof container. Melt the soap base into liquid form, then add the banana peel powder, French pink clay, carrier oil, and essential oil and mix. Pour this mixture into a recyclable/reusable container. Let the soap solidify for 12 to 15 hours, then cut it into bars.

Moringa Herby Soap Base

Shelf Life: This soap will last for 3 to 6 months.

Moringa is a plant we used to eat in India during monsoon season to detox our bodies and is a genuine wonder ingredient for the skin. It creates a high occlusive layer on bare surfaces and helps dermatitis, eczema, and psoriasis, revitalizes dry and dull skin, reduces fine wrinkles, and prevents the sagging of facial muscles. Moringa is also used in Ayurvedic medicine because it has antiseptic and anti-inflammatory properties. If you use moringa oil regularly, it will help reduce pimples and blemishes and brighten your skin tone!

The other star ingredient in this recipe is kale stem powder. This nutrient-packed leafy green is now used in everything from face masks to body lotions. Here are a few benefits of kale stem:

1. Kale is packed with antioxidants, which help protect the skin from damage caused by free radicals.
2. Kale is a great source of vitamins A, C, and E, which are essential for healthy skin.
3. The nutrient-rich nature of kale helps to nourish and revitalize the skin.

This soap works wonders on your body because it is made with oil, ensuring that your skin stays hydrated.

Ingredients

Phase	Amount	Role of Ingredient	Ingredients
Phase A	82% (82 ounces)	Foundational	Any vegan melt and pour soap base (coconut is my favorite)
Phase A	13% (13 ounces)	Functional	Kale stem powder (see Powdered Herbal Scraps on page 37)
Phase B	2% (2 ounces)	Additive	Parsley stem powder (see Powdered Herbal Scraps on page 37)

(continued on page 100)

Phase	Amount	Role of Ingredient	Ingredients
Phase B	2% (2 ounces)	Functional/utilitarian	Any lightweight carrier oil infused with any citrus peel
Phase B	1% (1 ounce)	Aromatic	Spearmint essential oil

Method

Cut your soap base into small pieces and add them to a heatproof container. Melt the soap base into liquid form, then add the powders, carrier oil, and essential oil and mix. Pour this mixture into a recyclable/reusable container. Let the soap solidify for 12 to 15 hours, then cut it into bars.

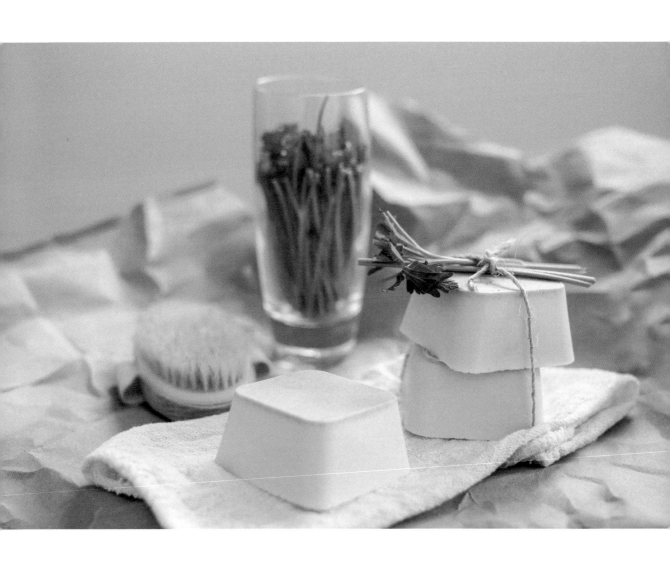

Nourishing Body Moisturizers

Homemade moisturizers can be made with the help of one or two affordable ingredients. Not only are they easy to make, but they also work better than more expensive products found at the drugstore. In making homemade body moisturizers, you have control over what goes into your products and can avoid using ingredients that may serve no purpose on the body, such as dyes and perfumes.

The best time to moisturize the skin is after a bath or shower. Doing so keep the skin moist, preventing bacteria, viruses, and irritants from entering the body. The following recipes will help you find the best body moisturizer for your skin type.

Body Oil for Dry Skin

Shelf Life: This oil will last for 3 to 6 months.

Body oil works wonders on the skin, especially dry skin. It promotes the skin's elasticity by making it soft, provided you use it regularly. This formula ensures that your body stays hydrated and smooth.

In this body oil, carrot peels are our superstar! They contain high levels of Vitamins A, C, and K, which are all essential for maintaining healthy skin. Vitamin A promotes cell turnover, while vitamin C brightens the skin and reduces inflammation. Vitamin K is important for helping the skin to heal and preventing bruises. In addition, carrot peels contain antioxidants that help protect the skin from damage caused by free radicals. If you are into ayurvedic therapies, you might know the importance of prewash body massage (abhyanga). All these benefits are mixed into this one beauty product to ensure that dry skin is a thing of the past.

Ingredients

Phase	Amount	Role of Ingredient	Ingredients
Phase A	1% (1 ounce)	Functional/utilitarian	Vitamin E
Phase A	1% (1 ounce)	Aromatic	Your favorite essential oil
Phase A	98% (98 ounces)	Foundational	Carrot peel–infused almond oil (see Infusions on page 41)

Method

In a bottle, add vitamin E and your favorite essential oil to the carrot peel–infused almond oil and shake well. Use this body oil when your body is slightly damp (directly after a bath or shower).

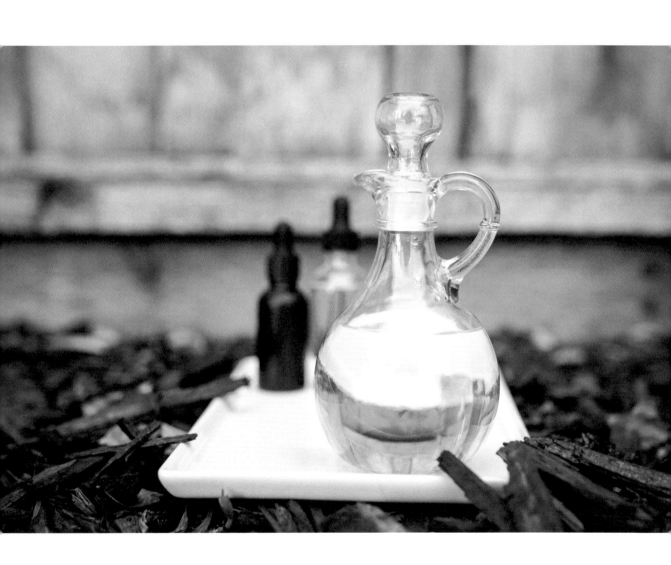

Body Oil for Oily Skin

Shelf Life: This body oil will last up to 6 months.

Using oil on oily skin—sounds weird, right? But trust me, by using the ingredients in the table below, you will not shy away from using oil on oily skin! Lemon peels can help prevent pores from becoming clogged. The citric acid in lemon peel helps to exfoliate the skin, removing dead skin cells and excess oil. In addition, lemon peel contains astringent properties that help tighten pores and control oil production. The biggest benefit of this lemon peel–infused body oil is its ability to penetrate the skin quickly without being oily on the skin's surface. For people with oily skin, this oil does not add to the existing problem. Instead, it solves it.

Ingredients

Phase	Amount	Role of Ingredient	Ingredients
Phase A	1% (1 ounce)	Functional/utilitarian	Vitamin E
Phase A	1% (1 ounce)	Aromatic	Your favorite essential oil
Phase A	98% (98 ounces)	Foundational	Lemon peel–infused grapeseed oil (see Infusions on page 41)

Method

In a bottle, add vitamin E and your favorite essential oil to the lemon peel–infused grapeseed oil and shake well. Massage this oil onto your body immediately after a bath or shower when your skin is still wet. Doing this will deliver nutrients to the skin and make it radiant.

Body Oil for Combination Skin

Shelf Life: This body oil will last up to 6 months.

If you are throwing away watermelon rinds, stop right there! Here are three reasons watermelon rinds are good for your skin:

1. They help balance your skin's pH levels.
2. They are packed with antioxidants and vitamins that help protect your skin from damage.
3. They are hydrating, which is important for maintaining healthy, glowing skin.

This formula treats inflammation on the skin and removes dark spots from the body and around the eyes. Its benefits do not end there. It also helps remove body acne, eczema, sunburns, and rashes.

Ingredients

Phase	Amount	Role of Ingredient	Ingredients
Phase A	98% (98 ounces)	Foundational	Watermelon rind–infused rice bran oil (see Infusions on page 41)
Phase A	1% (1 ounce)	Functional/utilitarian	Vitamin E
Phase A	1% (1 ounce)	Aromatic	Your favorite essential oil

Method

In a bottle, add vitamin E and your favorite essential oil to the watermelon rind–infused rice bran oil and shake well. Apply this oil to damp skin right after the bath or shower.

Minty Choco Body Butter for Dry Skin

Shelf Life: This body butter will last up to 6 months. Store it in a cool, dark place.

Anhydrous, water-free, or *waterless* refer to products that do not contain water. They use soothing botanical ingredients and nourishing oils to create a potent formula that diminishes the need for unnecessary fillers or preservatives. Some products are naturally water-free but most body lotions and creams found in a drugstore are not water-free. Some companies replace water with rose water and try to market it as water-free, but it is still water; the same goes for aloe vera gel, which contains 99.5 percent water. With this recipe, you can make your own water-free body butter. Mint stems are a hidden gem. The menthol in the mint stem can help soothe itchiness and dryness. In addition, mint stems can help relieve muscle aches and pains. Mint stem is also a great way to exfoliate your skin naturally. Mint stems' abrasive nature can help slough away dead skin cells, revealing brighter, more radiant skin. When infused with sunflower oil, then mixed with vitamin E, an antioxidant on its own, you can create a perfect product that protects your skin.

Ingredients

Phase	Amount	Role of Ingredient	Ingredients
Phase A	45% (45 ounces)	Foundational	Mint stem–infused sunflower oil (see Infusions on page 41)
Phase A	54% (54 ounces)	Functional/utilitarian	Cocoa butter
Phase B	1% (1 ounce)	Antioxidant	Vitamin E

Method

Use a double boiler or bain-marie to melt the oil and butter until fully molten. Set aside to cool. You can place the bowl in the fridge to speed up this process, but don't let it get rock-solid. Once firm, add in the vitamin E. Whisk to create a light, fluffy cream, then transfer to a jar with a lid.

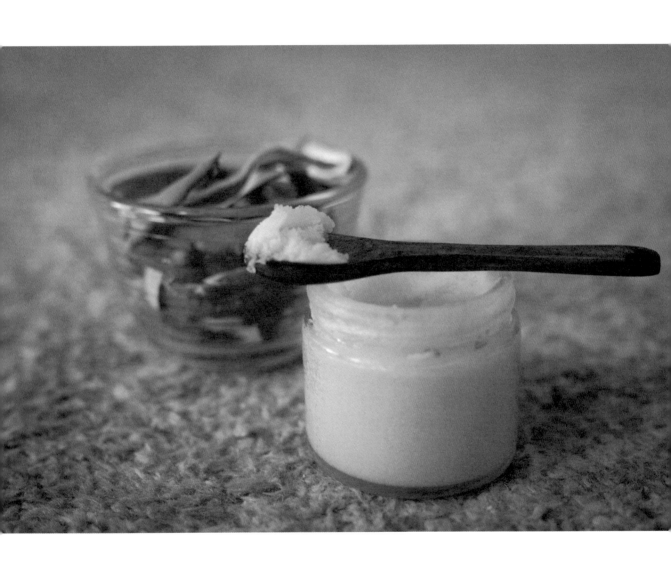

Lightweight Floral Body Butter for All Skin Types

Shelf Life: This body butter will last up to 6 months. Store it in a cool, dark place.

We all know sweet potatoes are delicious, but did you know they can also be good for your skin? Sweet potato peels are high in antioxidants, which help fight against free radicals that cause damage to the skin. Additionally, sweet potato peels are hydrating and can help reduce the appearance of fine lines and wrinkles. So, if you're looking for an antiaging skin-care solution, sweet potato peel may be just what you need! Try it and see for yourself. You'll be sure to see a difference in your skin's appearance.

Now, looking for a body butter that does it all? Say hello to murumuru butter! This Amazonian wonder butter is packed with fatty acids, vitamins, and minerals that nourish and condition the skin. It's also beautifully creamy and melts readily into the skin, making it ideal for body care. If you can't find this butter, you can swap it with mango butter.

Ingredients

Phase	Amount	Role of Ingredient	Ingredients
Phase A	45% (45 ounces)	Foundational	Sweet potato peel–infused almond oil (see Infusions on page 41)
Phase A	53% (53 ounces)	Functional/utilitarian	Murumuru butter
Phase B	1% (1 ounce)	Antioxidant	Vitamin E
Phase B	1% (1 ounce)	Aromatic	Geranium essential oil

Method

Use a double boiler or bain-marie to melt the oil and butter completely. Set aside to cool. You can place the bowl in the fridge to speed up this process, but don't let it get rock solid. Once firm, whisk to create a light, fluffy cream, then put it in the freezer. Take it out of the freezer after 5 to 10 minutes and whisk again. Add the vitamin E and essential oil, then transfer to a jar with a lid.

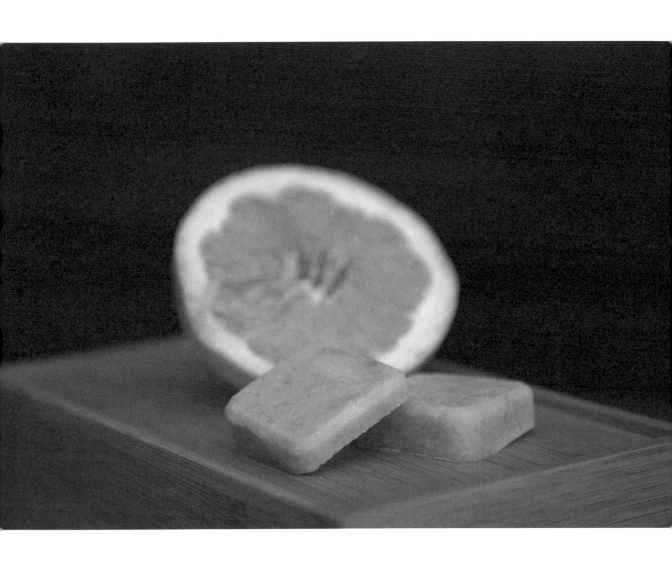

Exotic Citrusy Lotion Bar

Shelf Life: This lotion bar will last 10 to 12 months.

This exotic citrusy lotion bar is easy to make, eco-friendly, and sustains zero waste. It effectively gives the skin a fresh glow with ingredients like kokum butter, grapefruit peel–infused argan oil, mango butter, and vitamin E. These ingredients have antioxidant and anti-inflammatory properties that help keep the skin moist and free from irritation and wrinkles.

Ingredients

Phase	Amount	Role of Ingredient	Ingredients
Phase A	70% (44 ounces)	Foundational	Kokum butter
Phase A	20% (53 ounces)	Functional/utilitarian	Mango butter
Phase A	8% (1 ounce)	Functional/utilitarian	Grapefruit peel–infused argan oil (see Infusions on page 41)
Phase B	1% (1 ounce)	Antioxidant	Vitamin E
Phase B	1% (1 ounce)	Aromatic	Grapefruit essential oil

Method

Melt the butters in a double boiler or bain-marie. Remove from heat and let cool slightly, then add the argan oil and vitamin E. Finally, blend in the essential oil. Continue stirring until the mixture begins to solidify but is still pourable. Pour the mixture into soap molds or muffin molds and leave to set for 12 to 15 hours. Once solid, remove the bars from the molds and wrap them in parchment paper.

Woodsy Massage Oil

Shelf Life: This massage oil will last up to 4 months.

This formula combines apple peel–infused apricot kernel oil, kokum butter, vitamin E, and cinnamon or clove essential oil to soothe the skin and prevent acne, inflammation, and dryness on the skin. Not only are apples a renewable resource, but the peels are packed with nutrients that are great for your skin! Apple peel contains vitamin C, which is essential for collagen production, and it also has antioxidants that help protect your skin from damage. In addition, apple peel has astringent properties that can help tighten pores and improve skin texture.

Ingredients

Phase	Amount	Role of Ingredient	Ingredients
Phase A	19% (19 ounces)	Functional/utilitarian	Kokum butter
Phase A	79% (79 ounces)	Foundational	Apple peel–infused apricot kernel oil (see Infusions on page 41)
Phase B	1.75% (1.75 ounces)	Antioxidant	Vitamin E
Phase B	0.25% (0.25 ounce)	Aromatic	Cinnamon or clove essential oil

Method

Using a double boiler or bain-marie, melt the kokum butter on low heat. Once it's melted, stir in the apple peel–infused apricot kernel oil, vitamin E, and cinnamon or clove essential oil. Pour it into a pump jar and store in a cool, dark place.

Body Scrubs and Masks

Exfoliation removes dead skin cells from the surface of the skin. Body scrubs are one type of exfoliant, and they work by sloughing away dead skin cells with abrasive ingredients like salt, sugar, or coffee grounds. Body masks are another type of exfoliant, and they typically contain ingredients such as clay or cucumber that help hydrate and nourish the skin. While body scrubs can be used independently, body masks are usually applied after a scrub to help lock in moisture and nutrients.

Body exfoliation is important for several reasons. First, it improves circulation and promotes cell turnover. Second, it unclogs pores and prevents acne. Third, it evens out skin tone and texture. Exfoliating regularly can also help reduce the appearance of cellulite and stretch marks. There are many ways to exfoliate the body, but one of the most popular methods is ayurvedic gharshan. Gharshan is a Sanskrit word that means "to rub." It's an ancient Indian technique that uses a dry cloth to exfoliate the skin. The benefits of gharshan include improved circulation, better digestion, and deeper relaxation. Gharshan can be done on its own or as part of an ayurvedic massage. If you're interested in trying gharshan, use a gentle cloth and avoid scrubbing too hard, as this can irritate the skin.

You might think, why would I want to put a mask on my body? I already put a face mask on, isn't that enough? Well, let me tell you why body masks are important and why you should use them! Body masks are great for exfoliating your skin. They remove dead skin cells to reveal softer, smoother skin. In addition, body masks hydrate and nourish your skin. They also improve circulation and promote cell turnover.

Emulsified Pistachio Matcha Scrub

Shelf Life: This scrub is made to use. I recommend making right before taking a bath or shower.

This body scrub recipe is a good one to start with. Coconut oil contains linoleic acid and lauric acid, which are good for treating acne on the skin. They also have anti-inflammatory and antibacterial agents in their composition, making them useful in improving the texture of the skin and repairing skin defects. Pomegranate peel–infused avocado oil protects the skin from environmental toxins. When mixed with pistachio shell powder, an abrasive ingredient perfect for exfoliation, the result is a highly functional body scrub that cleanses the skin thoroughly and unclogs pores. This scrub also ensures that the skin stays hydrated throughout the day because it is oil-based.

Ingredients

Phase	Amount	Role of Ingredient	Ingredients
Phase A	5% (5 ounces)	Foundational	Coconut oil
Phase A	45% (45 ounces)	Foundational	Pomegranate peel–infused avocado oil (see Infusions on page 41)
Phase C	1% (1 ounce)	Additive	Vitamin E
Phase C	1% (1 ounce)	Aromatic	Matcha powder
Phase B	48% (48 ounces)	Functional/utilitarian	Pistachio shell powder (page 45)

Method

In a small heatproof bowl, add the coconut oil and pomegranate peel–infused avocado oil and melt thoroughly. Add in the vitamin E and matcha powder. Once submerged, slowly stir in the pistachio shell powder, and your scrub is ready to use. Start by applying the mix to your body. Leave the mix on for some minutes until it dries, then scrub gently and rinse off with lukewarm water. Pat your skin dry.

Salty Herbal Scrub

Shelf Life: This scrub is made to use. I recommend making right before taking a bath or shower.

This salty herbal scrub removes acne faster than other body scrubs for oily skin. Salt absorbs dirt and toxins from the body and cleanses the skin. Its mineral content keeps the skin hydrated, and its anti-inflammatory properties help treat irritation on the skin. Cilantro stem powder is rich in vitamins A and C and antioxidants that help prevent skin cell damage and remove wrinkles, sagging skin, and pigmentation of the skin. It also soothes irritation and kills infection on the skin. Cilantro stem powder is good for greasy skin and treats wounds sustained on the skin. Mint stem has antibacterial properties that make it a functioning body tone agent, moisturizer, and body cleanser. In addition, its anti-inflammatory properties help prevent acne on the body, especially for people with oily skin, and it also heals cuts, wounds, and itchy skin. Grapeseed oil moisturizes dull and dehydrated skin. It can tone the skin and reduce wrinkles on the body. Because of its vitamin E content, it also reduces the elasticity of the skin. All of these ingredients are combined in this recipe to ensure that your skin is evenly toned and well moisturized.

Ingredients

Phase	Amount	Role of Ingredient	Ingredients
Phase A	30% (30 ounces)	Foundational	Salt
Phase A	30% (30 ounces)	Foundational	Cilantro stem powder (see Powdered Herbal Scraps on page 37)
Phase A	40% (40 ounces)	Functional	Mint stem–infused grapeseed oil (see Infusions on page 41)

Method

Add salt and cilantro stem powder to a bowl. Slowly add in the mint stem–infused grapeseed oil and combine. To use, apply to wet skin and gently scrub in a circular motion. Rinse off with lukewarm water and pat your body dry with a towel. Apply a moisturizer or body oil to your body after use.

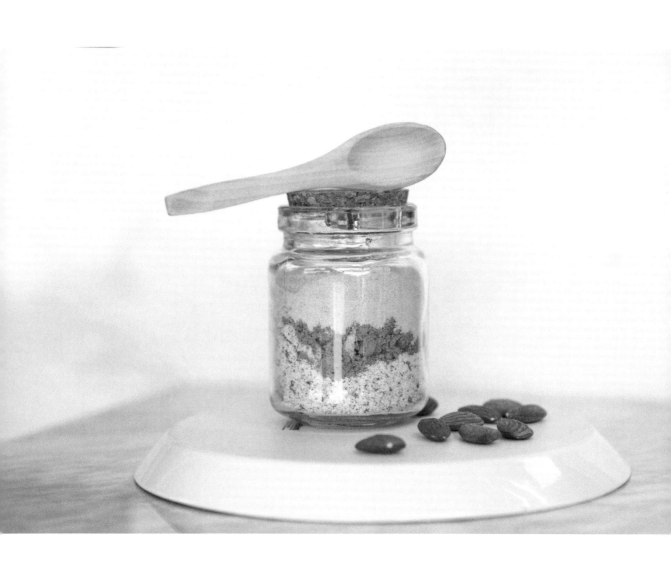

Dry Rub Almond-Turmeric Scrub

Shelf Life: This scrub is made to use. I recommend making right before taking a bath or shower.

This body scrub is made from three active ingredients: turmeric powder, orange peel powder, and ground almonds. When mixed together, they become a potent body scrub. Turmeric powder has anti-inflammatory agents for wound healing that occur on the skin. It also helps slow aging, as it has antioxidants that protect the skin from damage. Turmeric powder is good for treating cracked skin and removing stretch marks on the body. Its benefits do not end there; mixing turmeric powder with orange peel powder, an ingredient that helps brighten the skin because of its high citric acid content, gives the skin a fresh look while reducing scars, dark spots, and pigmentation. Like orange juice, orange peel powder is rich in vitamin C, which cleans pores and removes excess oil from the skin. I cannot fail to mention its antioxidant and anti-inflammatory properties that work on the skin to remove wrinkles, sagging skin, and inflammation. Ground almonds nourish and soften the skin and are rich in vitamin E. The combination of these products gives the skin a healthy tone and glow while healing scars, wrinkles, and dark spots on the body.

Ingredients

Phase	Amount	Role of Ingredient	Ingredients
Phase A	50% (50 ounces)	Foundational	Orange peel powder (see Powdered Herbal Scraps on page 37)
Phase B	45% (45 ounces)	Functional/utilitarian	Ground almonds
Phase A	5% (5 ounces)	Foundational	Turmeric powder

(continued on next page)

Method

This is the easiest body scrub to put together. Simply mix orange peel powder and ground almonds, then add in turmeric powder and mix once more. To use, apply on wet skin and gently scrub in a circular motion. Rinse off with lukewarm water and pat skin dry with a towel. Apply a moisturizer or body oil on your skin after use.

My Go-to Walnutty Soapy Scrub

Shelf Life: This scrub will last up to 1 month.

This soapy scrub helps deal with skin conditions like rashes, acne, irritation, and others. The mixture of castile soap and walnut shell powder forms an active body scrub. Grapefruit peel powder is rich in vitamin C and has antioxidants that tone the skin. The combination of these three ingredients produces a body scrub capable of dealing with all skin problems, including redness, acne, clogged pores, dark spots, and patches. This soapy scrub works well on oily skin.

Ingredients

Phase	Amount	Role of Ingredient	Ingredients
Phase A	10% (10 ounces)	Additive	Grapefruit peel powder (see Powdered Herbal Scraps on page 37)
Phase A	40% (40 ounces)	Functional	Walnut shell powder
Phase A	50% (50 ounces)	Foundational	Castile soap

Method

Mix the grapefruit peel powder and walnut shell powder together. Using a whisk, mix in the castile soap until a scrub-like texture forms. I recommend using this luxurious scrub once a week as a self-care ritual.

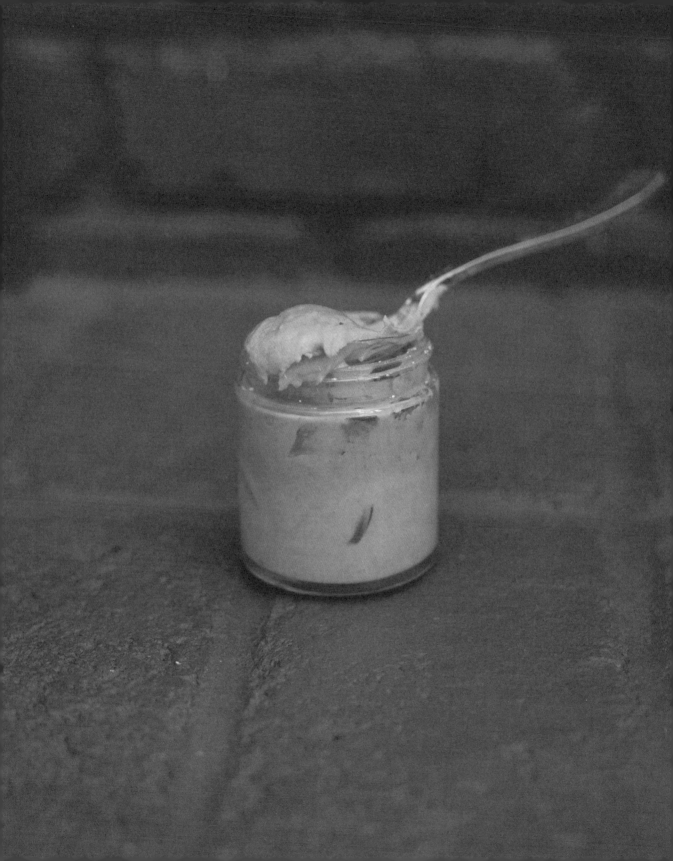

Turmeric Body Mask (Ubtan)

Shelf Life: This body mask is made to use.

In India, this body mask, a.k.a. ubtan, is applied to brides and grooms right before their wedding day. It's been said that this body mask will brighten brides' and grooms' skin on their wedding day. To create this product, you need chickpea flour, orange peel powder, and coconut oil. Chickpea flour reduces hyperpigmentation of the skin and ensures that the skin glows, especially the elbow, back of the neck, and armpit areas. Orange peel powder reduces pigmentation by removing spots on the body that can be caused by skin infections and sun exposure. Coconut oil helps keep the body hydrated if used immediately after your bath or shower. Combining these three ingredients gives you a body scrub that brightens your skin and gives it a glowing radiance free from wrinkles, acne, and eczema.

Ingredients

Phase	Amount	Role of Ingredient	Ingredients
Phase A	30% (30 ounces)	Foundational	Chickpea flour
Phase A	30% (30 ounces)	Foundational	Orange peel powder (see Powdered Herbal Scraps on page 37)
Phase A	40% (40 ounces)	Functional	Coconut oil, melted

Method

In a small bowl, mix the chickpea flour and orange peel powder and set aside. Then, slowly add the melted coconut oil to your dry mixture and combine. Apply this mask to your body and let it dry for 10 to 15 minutes. Rinse off with lukewarm water and pat your body dry. Make sure to moisturize your skin after use!

Mojito Body Mask

Shelf Life: This scrub is made to use. I recommend making right before taking a bath or shower.

This body mask removes acne, blemishes, dark spots, and dead skin. Rice flour is rich in anti-inflammatory and antioxidant properties, which reduce the sun's effects on the body, promote skin glow, and prevent the skin from aging quickly. Pineapple peel powder is rich in vitamin C and effective in fighting off bacteria on the skin's surface. Coconut oil gives you soft skin by ensuring that the body stays hydrated. It takes care of rashes, redness, acne, eczema, pimples, and irritation on the body.

Ingredients

Phase	Amount	Role of Ingredient	Ingredients
Phase A	30% (30 ounces)	Foundational	Rice flour
Phase A	30% (30 ounces)	Foundational	Pineapple peel powder (see Powdered Herbal Scraps on page 37)
Phase A	40% (40 ounces)	Functional	Coconut oil, melted

Method

In a small bowl, mix the rice flour and pineapple peel powder and set aside. Then, slowly add the melted coconut oil to your dry mixture and combine. Apply this mask to your body and let it dry for 10 to 15 minutes. Rinse off with lukewarm water and pat your body dry. Make sure to moisturize your skin after use!

Hand- and Foot-Care Recipes

Many of us spend hours trying to perfect our hair, makeup, and bodies. But what if I tell you that true beauty starts from the ground up? That's right. Taking care of your hands and feet is essential for sustainable beauty. Here's why:

For starters, your hands and feet are the most hardworking parts of your body. They're constantly exposed to the elements and take a lot of abuse daily, so it makes sense to give them some extra TLC. Plus, taking care of your hands and feet can improve your overall health. Many aestheticians and beauty enthusiasts express that regular hand and foot care can help improve circulation, reduce stress, and promote better sleep.

As a beauty addict myself, here are my tips for sustainable hand and foot care:

1. Exercise regularly. This helps increase blood flow and prevent stiffness and joint pain.
2. Eat a healthy diet. A balanced diet helps keep bones and muscles healthy.
3. Wear comfortable shoes. Shoes that fit well and support the feet can help prevent injuries.
4. Protect your skin. Wear sunscreen and avoid excessive sun exposure to prevent damage from ultraviolet rays.

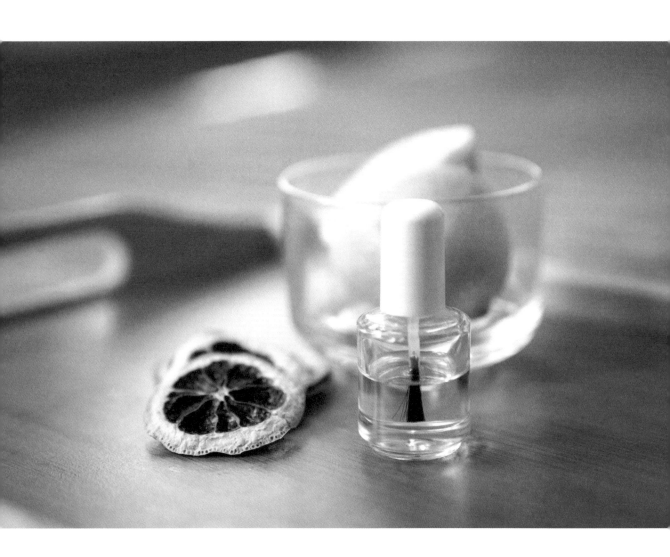

Wintery Cuticle Oil

Shelf Life: This oil will last up to 6 months.

Manicures and pedicures are great ways to take care of your nails, but there are so many other beneficial DIY nail products that you can incorporate into your sustainable beauty routine. The following nail-care products can be made from the comfort of your home and are sustainable and safe to use.

This wintery cuticle oil combats the harsh weather by moisturizing the hands and the nails. The lemon peel brightens the nails, and grapeseed oil reduces skin aging and keeps the skin smooth and soft. Paired with vitamin E, an ingredient rich in antioxidants, this cuticle oil is a potent product that is sure to take care of your nails during the winter months.

Ingredients

Phase	Amount	Role	Ingredients
Phase A	98% (98 ounces)	Foundational	Lemon peel–infused grapeseed oil (see Infusions on page 41)
Phase A	2% (2 ounces)	Functional/additive	Vitamin E

Method

Mix lemon peel–infused grapeseed oil with vitamin E and shake it well until the vitamin E is submerged in the grapeseed oil. Keep the bottle in a cool, dark place.

Hydra Cuticle Cream

Shelf Life: This cream will last up to 2 months.

This cuticle cream is great for summer nail care. Aloe vera gel acts as a humectant, which retains the moisture of cuticle skin. Paired with carrot peel–infused almond oil, this cuticle cream brightens the skin.

Ingredients

Phase	Amount	Role	Ingredients
Phase A	2% (2 ounces)	Functional	Carrot peel–infused almond oil (see Infusions on page 41)
Phase A	98% (48 ounces)	Foundational	Aloe vera gel

Method

Mix carrot peel–infused almond oil with aloe vera gel. Whisk until a cream-based consistency forms. If you are worried about dry skin near your cuticles, this cuticle cream is hydrating.

Store in a jar in a cool, dark place to reduce contamination. Apply the cream thinly to your nails three times a day.

Mint Choco Foot Balm

Shelf Life: This foot balm will last approximately 3 months.
Make sure not to expose it to any water.

If you have cracked heels or feel you are not doing enough to take care of your feet, don't worry, I've got you covered. This foot balm works like magic and is guaranteed to keep your skin hydrated and prevent it from becoming irritated or cracked, as it contains wax. Wax has moisturizing properties that work well for a dry and cracked heel. It can also help protect against dirt and debris, making it an ideal choice for those constantly on the go. Whether you're a runner, dancer, or simply someone who loves to walk, this foot balm will keep your feet feeling soft and healthy.

Ingredients

Phase	Amount	Role of Ingredient	Ingredients
Phase A	5% (5 ounces)	Foundational	Beeswax or any vegan wax
Phase A	45% (45 ounces)	Foundational	Cocoa butter
Phase B	48% (48 ounces)	Foundational	Mint stem–infused almond oil (see Infusions on page 41)
Phase C	1% (1 ounce)	Additive	Vitamin E
Phase C	1% (1 ounce)	Aromatic	Rose essential oil

Method

Gently melt the wax and butter in a double boiler or bain-marie. When melted, remove from heat and add in the mint stem–infused almond oil. Stir gently until it's about room temperature or you see a trace on the edges of the pot. Next, add the vitamin E and essential oil. Remember to stir until the liquid is still runny but turning more solid. Pour it into a wide-mouth jar and label the date. Apply this balm lightly to the cracked area of your feet before bed, then put on a clean sock.

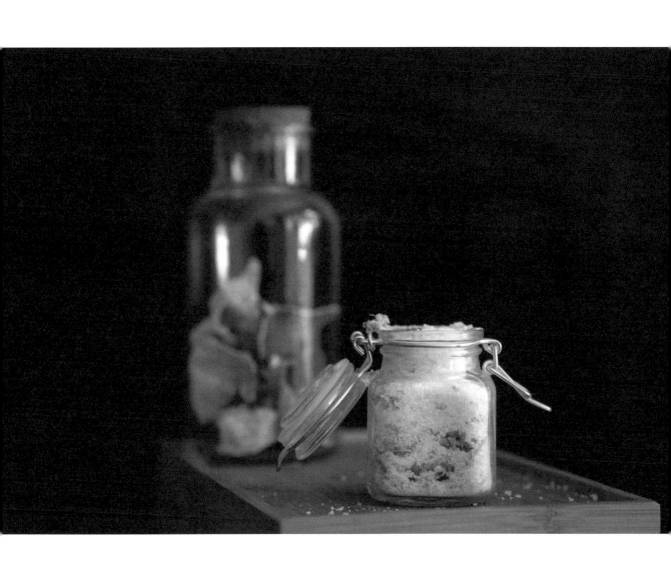

Orange Peel Foot Soak

Shelf Life: This foot soak will last approximately 6 months.
Make sure not to expose it to any water before use.

Whether you're looking to relax after a long day or pamper your feet before a pedicure, this foot soak is a great way to take care of feet! A foot soak is said to have many benefits, including stress relief, improved circulation, and detoxification. In this recipe, Epsom salt and orange peel work together as a scrubbing agent for the feet. Coconut milk powder soothes pain on the feet and makes dry skin soft. This foot soak can also help reduce foot odor.

Ingredients

Phase	Amount	Role of Ingredient	Ingredients
Phase A	30% (30 ounces)	Foundational	Epsom salt
Phase A	34% (34 ounces)	Foundational	Orange peel powder (see Powdered Herbal Scraps on page 37)
Phase B	34% (34 ounces)	Foundational	Coconut milk powder
Phase C	1% (1 ounce)	Additive	Vitamin E
Phase C	1% (1 ounce)	Aromatics	Orange essential oil

Method

To a jar with a lid, add the salt and powders and gently mix. Then, add the vitamin E and essential oil and mix once more. To use, fill your bathtub or foot tub up to ankle level with hot or warm water, then add three-quarters of this foot soak into the water. Soak your feet in the water for 10 to 15 minutes. Dry your skin thoroughly and moisturize your feet after use.

Walnutty Caffeinated Foot Scrub

Shelf Life: This foot scrub will last approximately 10 days in the fridge.
Make sure not to expose it to any water before use.

This foot scrub is effective for dry skin. Coffee grounds are beneficial to the skin because their rough texture exfoliates and removes dead skin cells. This foot scrub mixes coffee grounds with almond oil to provide a blend of exfoliation and moisturizing properties for the feet. Almond oil is great for massaging into the skin to prevent athlete's foot. Walnut shell powder provides toning functions for the skin and ensures that your skin becomes smoother and softer.

Ingredients

Phase	Amount	Role of Ingredient	Ingredients
Phase A	60% (60 ounces)	Foundational	Coffee ground–infused almond oil (see Infusions on page 41)
Phase A	40% (40 ounces)	Functional	Walnut shell powder

Method

To a jar with a lid, add all ingredients and gently mix until a thick paste is formed. To use, apply to wet feet and massage the feet for some minutes. Rinse off with lukewarm water, then dry and moisturize your feet immediately after use. I recommend applying this foot scrub once a week.

Cracked Heel Oil

Shelf Life: This oil will last approximately 3 months.
Store it in a dark cabinet and make sure not to expose it to the sun.

I love this recipe as I loved the minty smell of menthol from mint stems. To show your summer feet or make yourself ready to wear those summer flip-flops to the beach, this recipe is a fantastic solution for you to add to your body care regimen. This helps release stress and provides much needed hydration to heel those cracked feet.

Let me talk about the ingredients needed to make the cracked heel oil. First, you need shea butter. What shea butter does is that it acts as a moisturizing agent, and it makes the skin on the feet soft. It also has anti-inflammatory properties which help reduce redness on the skin and itchiness. Shea butter is rich in antioxidants, and it makes your skin elastic. The butter protects the feet from bacteria and ensures that the feet are smooth.

Another ingredient is apricot kernel oil infused with carrot peel. Using our food by-product along with goodies of apricot kernel oil. Apricot kernel oil is a good moisturizer for the skin and has anti-inflammatory properties. When infused with carrot peel, you have an ingredient capable of acting as an antiaging product that maintains the glow of the feet's skin. The last ingredient here is vitamin E pills or vitamin E. They have antioxidant properties. All these ingredients ensure that your feet are well moisturized and toned, and their elasticity is improved.

Ingredients

Phase	Amount	Role of Ingredient	Ingredients
Phase A	10% (10 ounces)	Foundational	Shea butter
Phase A	88% (88 ounces)	Functional/foundational	Carrot peel–infused apricot kernel oil (see Infusions on page 41)
Phase A	2% (2 ounces)	Additive	Vitamin E

(continued on next page)

Method

Using a double boiler or bain-marie, melt the shea butter on low heat. Add the melted shea butter to the carrot peel–infused apricot kernel oil and mix. Once the mixture is at room temperature, add in the vitamin E. Mix well and add mixture to a pump bottle. Apply this cracked heel oil to a bathtub or foot tub filled with warm water. Soak your feet in the water for 10 minutes and gently exfoliate your heels to remove any dirt, then remove your feet from the water and pat the skin dry. Apply moisturizer to your feet after use.

Chapter 7
Happy Hair Fixes

The following DIY recipes are good for your hair and the planet. Recipes include shampoos, conditioners, hair masks, scalp scrubs, dyes, rinses, and so much more! First, let's talk benefits of hair brushing.

Brushing your hair is essential for hair growth and hygiene. It flattens the outer layer of your hair shaft and makes it more reflective. In addition, it removes dirty deposits on the hair that can form together and breed bacteria and clog the pores on your scalp. It also moves oxygen and nutrients into the hair follicles by stimulating the capillaries of the scalp. Brushing your hair further functions as a hair conditioner that makes the hair strong, moisturized, smooth, and shiny.

No matter the hair you have, brushing makes it better. Brushes like the round-barrel brush are used for styling, while the paddle brush smooths the hair. In the same vein, the natural-bristle brush is versatile, and it smooths the hair. Make sure to remove hair from your brush after each use.

Hair Shampoos

How often should you shampoo your hair? It all depends on your hair type and scalp condition. For example, if you have dry hair, you might need to shampoo less often than someone with oily hair. And if you have a sensitive scalp, you might need to be careful about using harsh products. That's why I prefer DIY shampoos, so I know exactly what I am putting in my hair.

That said, a good rule of thumb is to shampoo every two to three days. This will help your scalp regulate its natural oil production and prevent your hair from looking greasy. If you feel you need to shampoo more often than that, do it, as you are the best judge of your hair. Be sure to use a gentle, DIY shampoo that won't strip your hair of its natural oils, and wash your hair in lukewarm water instead of hot water to prevent hair loss. Sustainable beauty is all about finding what works best for you and your hair to be consistent in your hair-care practices!

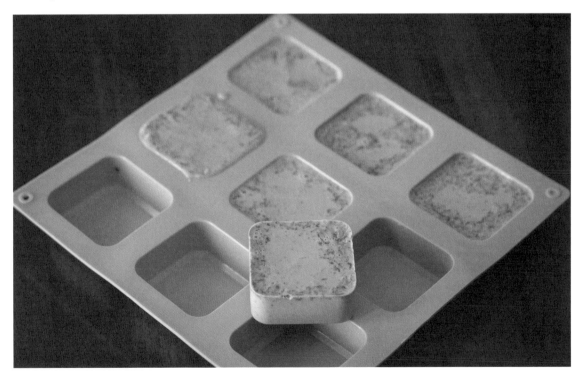

Ayurvedic Shampoo Powder

Shelf Life: This shampoo powder will last about 1 month. Make
sure it doesn't come into contact with water before use.

Ayurvedic shampoo powder makes the hair strong and healthy by cleansing and effectively preventing issues like dandruff, premature hair aging, and hair loss. Soapnut powder, also called shikakai powder, is rich in vitamins A, D, E, and K, which help make the hair smooth and shiny. Soapnut powder works well with all hair types and is an important ingredient for saponification. The efficacy of soapnut shampoo powder combined with fenugreek seed powder creates a fantastic hair product. Fenugreek can treat moderate hair loss in both men and women by helping with blood circulation, keeping the hair hydrated, and strengthening the roots of the hair. Rosemary stem powder also improves blood circulation, but its benefits do not end there; it takes care of the scalp's irritation, dryness, and dandruff while ensuring that the hair remains shiny.

Ingredients

Phase	Amount	Role of Ingredient	Ingredients
Phase A	50% (50 ounces)	Foundational	Soapnut powder
Phase A	45% (45 ounces)	Foundational	Fenugreek seed powder (see Powdered Herbal Scraps on page 37)
Phase A	5% (5 ounces)	Functional/utilitarian	Rosemary stem powder (see Powdered Herbal Scraps on page 37)

Method

This recipe calls for a good coffee grinder. Add soapnut powder to a coffee grinder and grind it smoothly, then add fenugreek seed powder and rosemary stem powder and grind one more time. Open the coffee grinder after 10 minutes and pack the shampoo powder in a jar with a lid. To apply this shampoo powder, mix with water. Massage thoroughly on hair and scalp and wash off.

Beetroot Ultra Hydrating Shampoo

Shelf Life: This shampoo will last about 1 month.

Beetroot is not only good for your heart and skin, but it can also do wonders for your hair! The carotenoids in beetroot help improve blood circulation to the scalp, which nourishes the hair follicles from within. In addition, the nutrients in beetroot (such as protein, vitamin A, and calcium) are essential for healthy hair growth.

This recipe contains the efficacy of beetroot with unscented castile soap, honey, and tea tree essential oil to make a powerful hair product. Castile soap is gentle on sensitive scalps and also effectively takes care of hair issues like dandruff, psoriasis, and dermatitis. Honey's humectant and emollient properties make the hair shiny and well moisturized. Honey can help prevent hair loss and breakage. Tea tree essential oil is also effective in preventing hair loss and removing dead skin, which help keep the hair healthy and strong.

Ingredients

Phase	Amount	Role of Ingredient	Ingredients
Phase A	85% (85 ounces)	Foundational	Unscented castile soap
Phase A	10% (10 ounces)	Foundational	Beetroot peel glycerite (see Glycerites on page 42)
Phase B	3% (3 ounces)	Functional/utilitarian	Honey
Phase B	2% (2 ounces)	Aromatic	Tea tree essential oil

Method

Using a small whisk, mix unscented castile soap with beetroot peel glycerite. Then, slowly add in the honey and essential oil and mix again. Store this shampoo in a pump bottle.

Green Shampoo Bars

Shelf Life: These shampoo bars will last 6 months.

Coconut oil serves as a protective barrier for the scalp by blocking damaging irritants and bacteria. Because coconut oil is rich in lauric acid, it nourishes your hair by getting absorbed into the hair strands, which keeps the hair moisturized and prevents it from breaking. Cilantro stem powder contains vitamins A, C, K, folic acid, riboflavin, and niacin. It does not just help hair growth; it cleanses the scalp and makes the hair shiny. Parsley stem powder is essential in hair care, as it improves blood circulation, promotes hair growth, and protects the hair from the effects of the sun. Rosemary essential oil has similar functions to parsley stem powder. It prevents the hair from turning grey early and works well against dandruff.

Ingredients

Phase	Amount	Role of Ingredient	Ingredients
Phase A	85% (85 ounces)	Foundational	Coconut oil soap base
Phase B	8% (8 ounces)	Functional/utilitarian	Cilantro stem powder (see Powdered Herbal Scraps on page 37)
Phase B	5% (5 ounces)	Functional/utilitarian	Parsley stem powder (see Powdered Herbal Scraps on page 37)
Phase B	2% (2 ounces)	Aromatic	Rosemary essential oil

Method

Cut the coconut oil soap base into small pieces and add them to a heatproof bowl. Melt the soap base into liquid form, then add both powders and the essential oil and mix. Pour this mixture into a recyclable/reusable container. Let the shampoo solidify for 12 to 15 hours, then cut it into bars.

Hair Conditioners

Have you ever wondered why your hair stylist always tells you to use conditioner, even if you have oily hair? Here's why: Conditioner helps protect your hair against the everyday environment, whether it's pollution or just the heat from hot water and styling tools. It means that your hair will experience less damage and look silky and shiny for longer. In addition, conditioner strengthens your hair by adding hydration and moisture. This is especially important in the winter when the air is cold and dry. Conditioner can help prevent your hair from becoming brittle and breaking. So, next time you're in the shower, don't skip the conditioner!

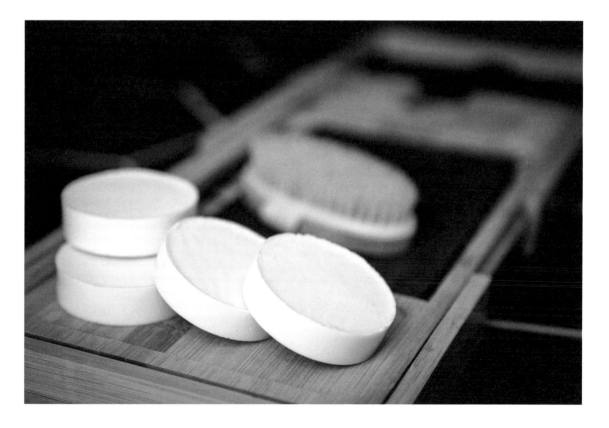

My Go-to Leave-in Conditioner

Shelf Life: This conditioner will last up to 6 months.

This leave-in conditioner is highly beneficial for every hair type. Both beetroot and pomegranate help improve blood circulation to the scalp and nourish the hair follicles. Rose water's vitamin A, B3, and E content ensures that the scalp is well moisturized and protected from heat and pollution. Rose water can also help prevent hair loss. Fractionated coconut oil is a moisturizing agent, and lemon peel is rich in vitamin C, which improves hair growth and reduces hair loss. It also cleanses the hair and scalp.

Ingredients

Phase	Amount	Role of Ingredient	Ingredients
Phase A	65% (65 ounces)	Foundational	Pomegranate peel or beetroot peel glycerite (see Glycerites on page 42)
Phase A	25% (25 ounces)	Functional/utilitarian	Rose water
Phase A	10% (10 ounces)	Functional/utilitarian	Lemon peel–infused fractionated coconut oil (see Infusions on page 41)

Method

Mix the glycerite and rose water, then slowly add in the infused oil and mix well. Store this mixture in a spray bottle. To use, shake well and apply to your washed, wet hair.

Creamy Co-washing Conditioner

Shelf Life: This conditioner will last for 2 months.
Keep water away from this product before use.

In simple terms, co-washing is the washing of hair using conditioners only. The primary significance of co-washing is that it does not have chemicals like sulphates that remove the hair's natural oils and cause breakage and dryness. Co-washing treats all types of hair textures without the use of shampoo.

Shea butter softens your hair, especially dry hair; repairs damage to the hair; revives hair follicles; and bolsters hair growth. Shea butter also makes the hair appear thicker and fuller. Rosemary stem–infused fractionated coconut oil is a two-in-one ingredient that moisturizes the hair, which makes it soft and helps prevents hair conditions like dandruff. Honey moisturizes the hair, improves hair growth, and prevents the hair from breaking. Aloe vera gel has vitamins A, B12, C, and E, amino acids, and fatty acids that strengthen the hair. It removes extra oil from the scalp of the hair and protects the hair and scalp from the adverse effects of sunlight. Vitamin B5 also protects the hair from the effects of the sun and keeps the hair hydrated and strong.

Ingredients

Phase	Amount	Role of Ingredient	Ingredients
Phase A	40% (40 ounces)	Foundational	Shea butter
Phase A	40% (40 ounces)	Functional/utilitarian	Rosemary stem–infused fractionated coconut oil (see Infusions on page 41)
Phase B	15% (15 ounces)	Functional/utilitarian	Honey or aloe vera gel
Phase B	5% (5 ounces)	Functional/utilitarian	Vitamin B5 powder

Method

Melt shea butter in a bowl and set aside. In a separate bowl, add the infused oil, honey or aloe vera gel, and vitamin B5 powder and mix until a creamy texture forms. Once the shea butter starts solidifying, add it into the creamy mixture and combine. Store in a bottle and use this conditioner for co-washing.

Hydrating Co-washing Conditioner

Shelf Life: This conditioner will last for 2 months.
Keep water away from this product before use.

Mango butter strengthens the hair follicles to give you firmer, smoother, and shinier hair. Grapeseed oil acts as a moisturizer for dry hair and scalp. Cilantro stem makes the hair shine and promotes hair growth. Honey moisturizes the hair, improves hair growth, and prevents the hair from breaking. Aloe vera gel has vitamins A, B12, C, and E, amino acids, and fatty acids that strengthen the hair. It removes extra oil from the scalp of the hair and protects the hair and scalp from the adverse effects of sunlight. Vitamin B5 also protects the hair from the effects of the sun and keeps the hair hydrated and strong. When combined with the ingredients described above, you get a product that rebuilds the hair.

Ingredients

Phase	Amount	Role of Ingredient	Ingredients
Phase A	40% (40 ounces)	Foundational	Mango butter
Phase A	40% (40 ounces)	Functional/utilitarian	Cilantro stem–infused grapeseed oil (see Infusions on page 41)
Phase B	15% (15 ounces)	Functional/utilitarian	Honey or aloe vera gel
Phase B	5% (5 ounces)	Functional/utilitarian	Vitamin B5 powder

Method

Melt the mango butter in a bowl and set aside. In a separate bowl, add the infused oil, honey or aloe vera gel, and vitamin B5 powder and mix until a creamy texture forms. Once the shea butter starts solidifying, add it into the creamy mixture and combine. Store in a bottle and use this conditioner for co-washing.

Choco Loco Conditioning Bars

Shelf Life: The conditioning bars will last for 3 months.

Cocoa butter serves as a beneficial conditioner. It soothes and moisturizes the hair and protects the scalp. Cilantro-infused plant oil is a two-in-one ingredient that helps hair growth and treats the scalp. Plant-based oils such as almond oil, avocado oil, coconut oil, grapeseed oil, corn oil, flax seed oil, soybean oil, rice bran oil, and others moisturize and improve the general well-being of the hair. Glycerin gives the soap base a natural humectant, making the hair remain fresh after washing. The combination of these ingredients results in shiny, well-protected hair.

Ingredients

Phase	Amount	Role of Ingredient	Ingredients
Phase A	40% (40 ounces)	Foundational	Cocoa butter
Phase A	40% (40 ounces)	Functional/utilitarian	Cilantro-infused plant oil of choice (see Infusions on page 41)
Phase B	15% (15 ounces)	Functional/utilitarian	Cilantro stem powder (see Powdered Herbal Scraps on page 37)
Phase B	5% (5 ounces)	Functional/utilitarian	Glycerin soap base, grated and melted

Method

This is the simplest conditioner bar you can make for yourself. First, melt the cocoa butter and infused oil using a double boiler or bain-marie. Once the mixture cools, add the cilantro stem powder and soap base. Pour this mixture into an ice cube tray and let it set at room temperature for 24 hours. Once set, take out the bars and store in a jar.

Hair and Scalp Scrubs and Masks

Regular scalp care is necessary if you're looking for long, luscious locks. A good scrub or mask will remove all the built-up gunk from your scalp, unclog hair follicles, and leave your hair looking and feeling healthier. Hair masks improve the condition of the hair by deep conditioning the hair, stimulating hair growth.

Not sure how to get started? Here are my top tips for incorporating hair scrubs and masks into your hair-care routine:

1. Use a hair scrub or mask once a week.
2. Apply the hair scrub or mask to dry hair before shampooing.
3. Focus on your scalp, not your hair, when applying the product.
4. Rinse thoroughly and follow up with your regular hair-care routine.

Now, let's get back to the recipes!

Pomegranate Floral Hair Scrub

Shelf Life: This scrub will last up to 12 months.

Are you dealing with split ends? This hair scrub has got you covered. Pomegranates contain a moisture sealant called ellagic acid, meaning no more greasy roots or dry ends between washes if used regularly (just like magic!), so you can have healthier strands without worrying about split ends ever again. Salt is a potent beauty care product that works wonders for the hair and skin. It supports a healthy scalp by removing dandruff particles and prevents oily hair by regulating the release of oil from the sebaceous glands to the scalp. Rose water moisturizes the hair and scalp and deals effectively with the effect of heat and pollution. Because of its anti-inflammatory properties, it also prevents conditions like eczema on the scalp.

Ingredients

Phase	Amount	Role of Ingredient	Ingredients
Phase A	60% (60 ounces)	Foundational	Sun-dried pomegranate peel powder (see Powdered Herbal Scraps on page 37)
Phase A	20% (20 ounces)	Functional/utilitarian	Table salt or Epsom salt
Phase B	20% (20 ounces)	Functional/utilitarian	Rose water

Method

Combine the sun-dried pomegranate peel powder and salt in a small jar. Mix this dry powder with rose water when ready for a hair wash. I recommend 20 ounces of rose water, but you can add more or less based on your preferences. Apply this mixture to your scalp and rub it in. Rinse and follow with a natural shampoo (see on page 134).

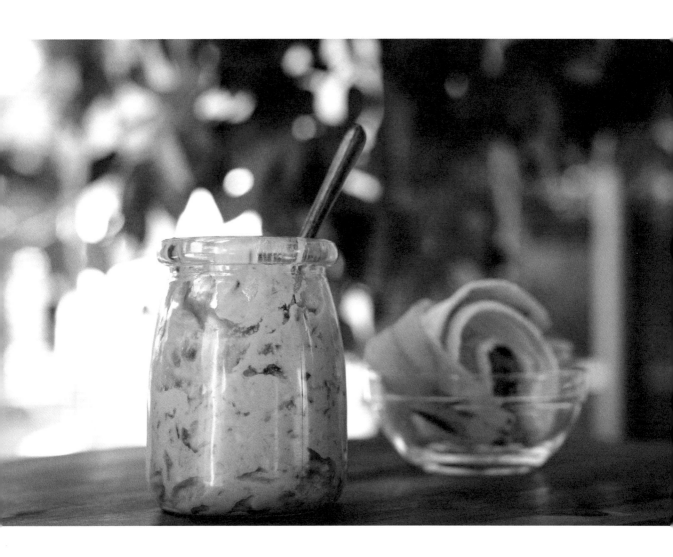

Avocado Banana Peel Hair Mask

Shelf Life: This mask is made to use.

Banana peels are not just for monkeys anymore! This green beauty hack has been gaining popularity as a natural hair-care solution. The nutrients in banana peels, including vitamins A, B, and C, boost hair growth and reduce dandruff. You can simply rub a banana peel on your scalp for a few minutes and rinse with shampoo or add a mashed banana peel to your regular shampoo or conditioner, but this hair mask is my all-time favorite to help with dandruff. Cilantro works wonders on the hair because it contains a rich source of vitamins and proteins that the hair needs to grow and shine. Avocado oil moisturizes the scalp, detangles and prevents hair breakage, and protects hair from the negative effects of pollution, sunlight, and chlorine. Greek yogurt is efficient in taming unruly hair strands, softening the hair, and treating dandruff. The combination of these ingredients results in this potent hair-care product.

Ingredients

Phase	Amount	Role of Ingredient	Ingredients
Phase A	60% (60 ounces)	Foundational	Mashed banana peel
Phase A	20% (20 ounces)	Functional/utilitarian	Cilantro-infused avocado oil (see Infusions on page 41)
Phase A	20% (20 ounces)	Functional/utilitarian	Greek yogurt

Method

Add all ingredients to a food processor and blend until a nice paste forms. Apply this hair mask once a week for thirty minutes before you wash your hair.

Emulsified Salty Hair and Scalp Scrub

Shelf Life: This scrub will last up to 15 days in the fridge.

Cucumbers are a great way to get your daily dose of vitamins C and K. They also contain plenty of silicon, calcium, sodium, etc., all vital for healthy hair growth! Castile soap works well on sensitive scalps and prevents dandruff, psoriasis, and dermatitis by keeping your hair and scalp hydrated. Salt gives the hair a healthy texture, makes it thicker, and clears blocked pores on the scalp.

Ingredients

Phase	Amount	Role of Ingredient	Ingredients
Phase A	50% (50 ounces)	Foundational	Unscented castile soap
Phase A	30% (30 ounces)	Functional/utilitarian	Epsom salt or table salt
Phase A	20% (20 ounces)	Functional/utilitarian	Sun-dried cucumber peel powder (see Powdered Herbal Scraps on page 37)

Method

Add the unscented castile soap, salt, and sun-dried cucumber peel powder to a large mixing bowl. Apply this hair and scalp scrub right to dry hair before taking a bath or shower, then rinse out and wash your hair with natural shampoo and conditioner.

Powdered Ayurvedic Hair Mask

Shelf Life: This mask has a longer shelf life of 3 to 6 months.

Rhassoul clay, found only in a valley in the Atlas Mountains in Morocco, has been used on the hair and skin for centuries. What makes this clay different from other types is that it contains silica, which works as an exfoliant for the hair, making it shiny, smooth, and soft. Amla powder is an ayurvedic ingredient used for centuries to treat various conditions like diarrhea, jaundice, and others. The benefit of amla powder on the hair is immeasurable. It helps in cleansing the scalp, promoting hair growth, improving the volume of hair, and treating dandruff and lice.

Ingredients

Phase	Amount	Role of Ingredient	Ingredients
Phase A	30% (30 ounces)	Foundational	Rhassoul clay
Phase A	20% (20 ounces)	Functional/utilitarian	Orange peel powder (see Powdered Herbal Scraps on page 37)
Phase A	20% (20 ounces)	Functional/utilitarian	Lemon peel powder (see Powdered Herbal Scraps on page 37)
Phase A	20% (20 ounces)	Functional/utilitarian	Amla powder
Phase A	10% (10 ounces)	Functional/utilitarian	Fenugreek seed powder (see Powdered Herbal Scraps on page 37)

Method

Add all ingredients to a large mixing bowl and combine. Store this mixture in an airtight container in a cool, dark place. Whenever you want to apply this hair mask, add water 3 tablespoons of water to 2 tablespoons of powder and mix. Add more or less water to reach your desired consistency. This is my go-to recipe when traveling because it contains mixed powders, which are easy to carry.

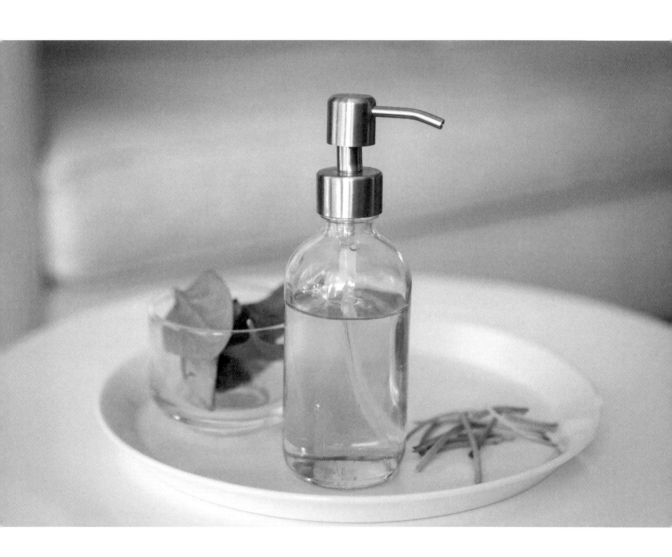

Overnight Hair Mask

Shelf Life: This mask will last up to 1 week.

Spinach stems are rich in vitamins A, B, C, and K, iron, magnesium, and zinc manganese that work together to ensure the hair has accelerated growth. Rosemary stem–infused oil has rich antioxidant and anti-inflammatory properties. It promotes blood circulation to the scalp, effectively preventing hair loss. It also enhances hair growth and prevents dandruff, itchy scalp, and premature graying. With the help of its antibacterial qualities, it also cleanses the hair thoroughly.

Ingredients

Phase	Amount	Role of Ingredient	Ingredients
Phase A	95% (95 ounces)	Foundational	Spinach stem glycerite (see Glycerites on page 42)
Phase A	5% (5 ounces)	Functional/utilitarian	Rosemary stem–infused oil of choice (see Infusions on page 41)

Method

To a small mixing bowl, add both ingredients and whisk well. Apply this mixture to your hair ends and scalp. This is an overnight hair mask, meaning you can apply this mixture at night and sleep with it on. Make sure you wear a shower cap to bed, as glycerite can be sticky. The next day, rinse out and wash your hair with natural shampoo and conditioner.

Nutty Hair Scrub

Shelf Life: This scrub is made to use.

This hair scrub effectively prevents skin irritation and frees your hair of excess oil. Walnut shell powder strengthens the hair because it is rich in potassium, omega-3, omega-6, and omega-9 fatty acids. It protects the hair from environmental pollution and the effects of sunlight, reduces hair loss, and helps fight dandruff and skin irritation. Pistachio shell powder stimulates hair growth by strengthening and deeply nourishing the hair. It works particularly well for dry hair. Pistachio shell powder also includes biotin, an agent that helps prevent hair loss. Lemon-infused glycerite makes the hair soft and smooth while cleansing it and the scalp.

Ingredients

Phase	Amount	Role of Ingredient	Ingredients
Phase A	60% (60 ounces)	Foundational	Walnut shell powder
Phase A	20% (20 ounces)	Functional/utilitarian	Pistachio shell powder
Phase B	20% (20 ounces)	Functional/utilitarian	Lemon Peel Glycerite (page 44)

Method

Add the powders to a large mixing bowl and combine. Store in a small jar in a cool, dark place. Whenever you want to apply this hair scrub, add 20 ounces of lemon peel glycerite to the powders and mix.

Sweet and Lovely Hair Mask

Shelf Life: This mask is made to use.

Amla powder works wonders on the hair by cleansing the hair and scalp of dirt and excess oil. The vitamin C in amla powder promotes hair growth, prevents the hair from smelling, and removes germs that stick to the hair while maintaining the color of the hair. Sweet potato peel moisturizes the hair and can aid in preventing hair loss. Rose water washes excess oil away from its scalp, keeps the hair hydrated, reduces the effects of pollution and sunlight on the hair, and makes the hair soft. Ultimately, rose water reduces stress, and stress is a major cause of hair loss.

Ingredients

Phase	Amount	Role of Ingredient	Ingredients
Phase A	30% (30 ounces)	Foundational	Amla powder or gooseberry powder
Phase A	30% (30 ounces)	Functional/utilitarian	Sweet Potato Peel Powder (page 44)
Phase A	40% (40 ounces)	Functional/utilitarian	Rose water

Method

Add the powders to a large mixing bowl, then slowly add rose water and mix until there are no lumps in the end product. To use, apply this hair mask to a brush and brush through your hair. Keep this mask on for 30 to 40 minutes, then rinse and wash your hair with natural shampoos and conditioners.

Water-Free Hair Mask

Shelf Life: This mask will last up to 1 month. For more of
a spa-like experience, store in the fridge and apply cold.

Rice flour has para-aminobenzoic acid, ferulic acid, and allantoin properties that make it a potent ingredient for beautiful hair and skin. It removes excess oil and dirt from the hair, repairs hair damage, and prevents more breakage. Lemon peel powder is rich in vitamin C, which helps improve the growth rate of the hair and increase the production of collagen around the hair. It's also rich in citric acid, which tightens the hair follicles and prevents hair loss. Lemon peel–infused almond oil makes your hair soft and easy to style. It also includes a high amount of vitamin E, which prevents stress around the hair, reduces hair loss, and strengthens the hair. Almond oil is removes excess oil from the scalp, which prevents dandruff and skin irritation.

Ingredients

Phase	Amount	Role of Ingredient	Ingredients
Phase A	40% (40 ounces)	Foundational	Rice flour
Phase A	30% (30 ounces)	Functional/utilitarian	Lemon peel powder (see Powdered Herbal Scraps on page 37)
Phase A	30% (30 ounces)	Functional/utilitarian	Lemon peel–infused almond oil (see Infusions on page 41)

Method

To a large mixing bowl, add the rice flour and lemon peel powder, then slowly add the lemon peel–infused almond oil and mix until a paste forms. If the consistency seems too dry, add more infused oil. Store in a small jar with a lid.

Hydrating Hair Mask

Shelf Life: This mask is made to use.

This mask is a quick fix for when my hair is feeling a little dull and I don't have any exotic ingredients on hand.

Ingredients

Phase	Amount	Role of Ingredient	Ingredients
Phase A	40% (40 ounces)	Foundational	Mashed avocado
Phase A	30% (30 ounces)	Functional/utilitarian	Avocado seed powder (see Powdered Herbal Scraps on page 37)
Phase A	30% (30 ounces)	Functional/utilitarian	Greek yogurt

Method

In a large mixing bowl, add the mashed avocado and avocado seed powder. Slowly add the Greek yogurt and mix until a paste forms. Apply this hair mask for thirty minutes before you wash your hair.

The Role of Hair Dye

Synthetic hair dyes are full of harsh chemicals that can damage your hair, especially if you dye it regularly. The chemicals in hair dye can strip away the natural oils that protect your hair, leaving it dry and brittle. They can also penetrate the hair shaft and damage the follicles, leading to thinning hair or baldness. If you're concerned about your hair's health, the following natural hair dye recipes are gentle on your hair and will cause no long-term damage.

Henna is an organic product with lots of cultural and medicinal value. The word henna is Arabic, but it is used for hair- and skin-care in India as an ayurvedic ingredient. Henna improves hair growth, reduces hair loss, conditions the hair, and prevents dandruff and itchiness. Henna works on all hair colors, but especially dark hair, as it enhances auburn and brown hair tones.

Overall, henna can be a good choice for those looking for a natural alternative to chemical hair dyes. However, it's essential to know the potential disadvantages before using. Henna can stain your skin orange if you accidentally apply it to your skin. Some people may be allergic to henna, which can cause symptoms like itching, redness, and swelling. Doing a patch test before using henna can help prevent these symptoms.

Henna Hair Dye, a.k.a Ayurvedic Hair Dye 1

Shelf Life: This hair dye is made to use and will last for 3–4 weeks once applied.

Making an ayurvedic hair dye with just henna might turn your hair orange or a non-desirable color. This recipe mixes henna with complementary ingredients like amla powder, fenugreek seed powder, and coffee grounds to yield a beautiful hair dye. Henna powder can produce an essential oil that nourishes the hair and promotes growth. Henna also reduces hair loss and serves as a deep conditioning agent for the hair. It protects the scalp of the hair and prevents dandruff and irritation that may occur on the scalp. In addition, if you want thicker hair, henna will do that for you while ensuring that your hair stays soft and shiny.

Amla powder cleanses the hair and scalp from dirt and excess oil. It prevents the hair from smelling because of its antimicrobial properties, prevents the hair from turning grey early, and makes the hair thick. Fenugreek seed powder ensures that the hair is hydrated, makes the root of the hair strong, and improves blood circulation to the hair.

As any sustainable beauty lover knows, coffee is a fantastic ingredient for hair care. Not only does it contain antioxidants that help protect the hair from damage, but it also contains caffeine, which stimulates the hair roots and follicles, helps reduce hair loss, and promotes growth. Plus, it imparts a rich brown color to the hair, making it a perfect natural dye.

Ingredients

Phase	Amount	Role of Ingredient	Ingredients
Phase A	40% (40 ounces)	Foundational	Henna powder
Phase A	10% (10 ounces)	Functional/utilitarian	Amla powder
Phase A	5% (5 ounces)	Functional/utilitarian	Fenugreek seed powder (see Powdered Herbal Scraps on page 37)
Phase B	45% (45 ounces)	Functional	Used coffee grounds

(continued on next page)

Method

In a large mixing bowl, add the henna powder, amla powder, and fenugreek seed powder. Mix and store in an airtight container. To complete this dye, submerge used coffee grounds in boiling water for 5 to 7 minutes. After the water cools down and the coffee grounds settle at the bottom, add the coffee ground–infused water to the powders and mix until a thick paste forms. Set paste aside overnight and apply to your hair the next day. After 3 to 4 hours, rinse out and wash your hair with a natural conditioner. Don't use shampoo.

Henna Hair Dye, a.k.a Ayurvedic Hair Dye 2

Shelf Life: This hair dye is made to use and will last for 3–4 weeks once applied.

Henna powder can produce an essential oil that nourishes the hair and promotes growth. Henna also reduces hair loss and serves as a deep conditioning agent for the hair. It protects the scalp of the hair and prevents dandruff and irritation that may occur on the scalp. In addition, if you want thicker hair, henna will do that for you while ensuring that your hair stays soft and shiny.

Amla powder cleanses the hair and scalp from dirt and excess oil. It prevents the hair from smelling because of its antimicrobial properties, prevents the hair from turning grey early, and makes the hair thick. Fenugreek seed powder ensures that the hair is hydrated, makes the root of the hair strong, and improves blood circulation to the hair.

Onion peel is perfect for people with dull hair and/or hair loss by ensuring that your hair does not break.

Ingredients

Phase	Amount	Role of Ingredient	Ingredients
Phase A	30% (30 ounces)	Foundational	Henna powder
Phase A	20% (20 ounces)	Functional/utilitarian	Amla powder
Phase A	10% (10 ounces)	Functional/utilitarian	Fenugreek seed powder (see Powdered Herbal Scraps on page 37)
Phase B	40% (40 ounces)	Functional	Onion peels

(continued on page 161)

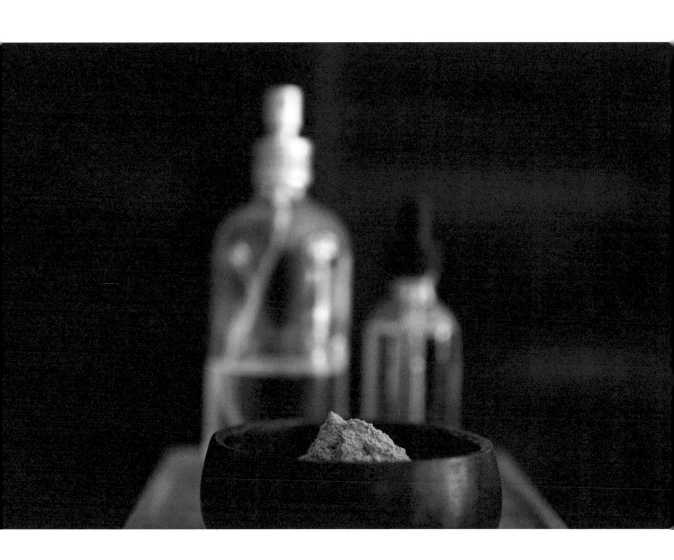

Method

Add henna powder, amla powder, and fenugreek seed powder to a large mixing bowl. Mix it well and store in an airtight container. To complete this dye, submerge onion peels in 32 ounces of boiling water. After the water cools down, discard the onion peels, add the onion peel–infused water to the powders, and mix until a thick paste forms. Set paste aside overnight and apply to your hair the next day. After 3 to 4 hours, rinse out and wash your hair with a natural conditioner. Don't use shampoo.

The Importance of Hair Oil

Not only does hair oil protect our heads from the elements, but it also plays a significant role in how we look and feel. Hair oil helps restore vitamins and minerals that can be stripped away by using detergent-based shampoos. It can also help protect against breakage and frizz and give damaged strands a polished and shiny appearance.

One of the best ways to apply hair oil is with the hot towel spa method, in which the hair is covered with a hot, damp towel after application. The practice of pouring oil into your hair and massaging it on the hair and scalp will also do wonders for your hair. It is highly recommended in ayurvedic medicine and has spread outside of ayurvedic medicine. Oiling the hair protects the hair from tearing, reduces the chances of having dry and swollen hair, and ensures that you have a healthy scalp. I recommend using plant-based oils like coconut oil, sesame oil, almond oil, argan oil, moringa oil, amla oil, and others.

If you want to keep your hair looking its best, use hair oil weekly. Your hair will thank you for it!

Cilantro Steamy Oil

Shelf Life: This oil will last for 3 months. Keep away from sunlight.

If you're struggling with dandruff or an itchy scalp, this cilantro steamy oil can help. Cilantro is known for its ability to improve circulation, which promotes a healthy scalp and cilantro stems make hair softer and more manageable. Argan oil, also known as liquid gold, is extracted from the kernels of the argan tree in Morocco. It has been used for cooking, health, and beauty purposes for centuries. It works wonders on the skin and the hair. It contains fatty acids and vitamin E, which moisturize hair and the scalp and prevent breakage.

Ingredients

Phase	Amount	Role of Ingredient	Ingredients
Phase A	100% (100 ounces)	Foundational	Cilantro stem–infused argan oil (see Infusions on page 41)

Method
Use this oil on the hair weekly.

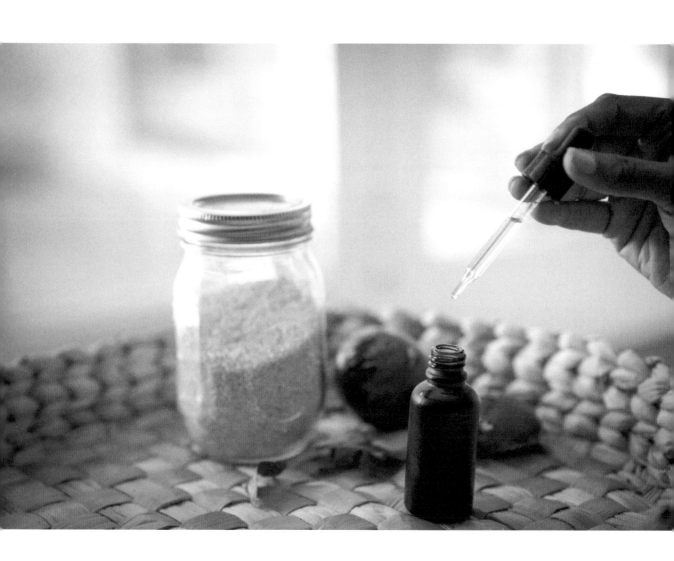

Sesame Hair Oil

Shelf Life: This oil will last for 3 months. Keep away from sunlight.

Sesame oil is a natural emollient for the hair that fights against dandruff, hair irritation, and negative effects of the sun. Coconut oil protects the hair because of its rich chemical composition. Onion peels prevent hair loss and dull and/or graying hair. Mint stem prevents hair loss by increasing blood circulation to the scalp. Mint stem–infused apricot kernel oil reduces excess dryness on the scalp, strengthens the hair, and promotes hair growth. Shea butter moisturizes the hair and makes it shine due to its vitamin A, E, and fatty acid content.

Ingredients

Phase	Amount	Role of Ingredient	Ingredients
Phase A	30% (30 ounces)	Foundational	Sesame oil
Phase A	30% (30 ounces)	Foundational	Onion peel–infused coconut oil (see Infusions on page 41)
Phase A	10% (10 ounces)	Foundational	Shea butter
Phase A	30% (30 ounces)	Foundational	Mint stem–infused apricot kernel oil (see Infusions on page 41)

Method

Add the sesame oil, onion peel–infused coconut oil, and shea butter to a double boiler or bain-marie. Once shea butter is melted, set the melted mixture aside. Slowly add in the mint stem–infused apricot kernel oil and mix. Store this hair oil in a glass bottle. Apply to unwashed hair and let it sit for 30 minutes before rinsing off. Follow with a hair wash.

Hydrating Oil for Hair Growth

Shelf Life: This oil will last for 3 months. Keep away from sunlight.

Both castor oil and orange peels improve blood circulation to the scalp to promote hair growth. Almond oil prevents hair breakage and works as an emollient to make the hair smooth, soft, and shiny. Coconut oil protects hair from the negative effects of the sun while ensuring that the hair remains soft and smooth.

Ingredients

Phase	Amount	Role of Ingredient	Ingredients
Phase A	40% (40 ounces)	Foundational	Castor oil
Phase A	30% (30 ounces)	Foundational	Orange peel–infused almond oil (see Infusions on page 41)
Phase A	30% (30 ounces)	Foundational	Coconut oil, liquid at room temperature

Method

Add all ingredients to a small glass bottle and shake well. Store in a cool, dark place. Apply this hair oil to unwashed hair and let it sit for 30 minutes, then rinse it out and wash your hair.

Fruity Hair Balm a.k.a Thick Oil

Shelf Life: This oil will last for 6 months.

Grapefruit makes the hair shiny because, as a citric fruit, it contains vitamins A and C, which help brighten the hair and cleanse the hair and scalp. Argan oil, also known as liquid gold, is extracted from the kernels of the argan tree in Morocco. It has been used for cooking, health, and beauty purposes for centuries. It works wonders on the skin and the hair. It contains fatty acids and vitamin E, which moisturize hair and the scalp and prevent breakage. Orange peels improve blood circulation to the scalp to promote hair growth. Almond oil prevents hair breakage and works as an emollient to make the hair smooth, soft, and shiny. Beeswax is rich in vitamin A and antibiotic agents that moisturize the hair and treat eczema, dandruff, and psoriasis.

Ingredients

Phase	Amount	Role of Ingredient	Ingredients
Phase A	40% (40 ounces)	Foundational	Grapefruit–infused argan oil (see Infusions on page 41)
Phase A	30% (30 ounces)	Foundational	Orange peel–infused almond oil (see Infusions on page 41)
Phase A	30% (30 ounces)	Functional	Beeswax or any vegan wax

Method

To a double boiler or bain-marie, add all ingredients and keep stirring until the wax is melted properly. Once the wax has totally melted, add to a tin container, and refrigerate until the balm has solidified a little bit. Keep this container in a cool, dark place. Apply this product to your unwashed hair and leave on for 30 minutes, then rinse off and wash your hair.

Two Ingredient Oil

Shelf Life: This oil will last for 3 months. Keep away from sunlight.

Rosemary stems have rich antioxidant and anti-inflammatory properties that promote blood circulation to the scalp, which help prevent hair loss, dandruff, itchy scalp, and premature greying. Argan oil, also known as liquid gold, is extracted from the kernels of the argan tree in Morocco. It has been used for cooking, health, and beauty purposes for centuries. It works wonders on the skin and the hair. It contains fatty acids and vitamin E, which moisturize hair and the scalp and prevent breakage. Vitamin E also acts as a protective layer for the scalp that keeps the hair moisturized.

Ingredients

Phase	Amount	Role of Ingredient	Ingredients
Phase A	98% (98 ounces)	Foundational	Rosemary stem–infused argan oil (see Infusions on page 41)
Phase	2% (2 ounces)	Functional	Vitamin E

Method

Combine the rosemary stem–infused argan oil with the vitamin E. Store in a glass bottle and use this hair oil once a week right before your hair wash.

Hair Rinses

Hair rinses are some of the most neglected hair-care products on the market, but they are a fantastic way to give your hair an extra dose of superfoods without adding any harsh ingredients. Hair rinses are great for people who are dealing with lifeless, damaged, and dull hair. Add the following hair rinse recipes to your at-home hair-care routine!

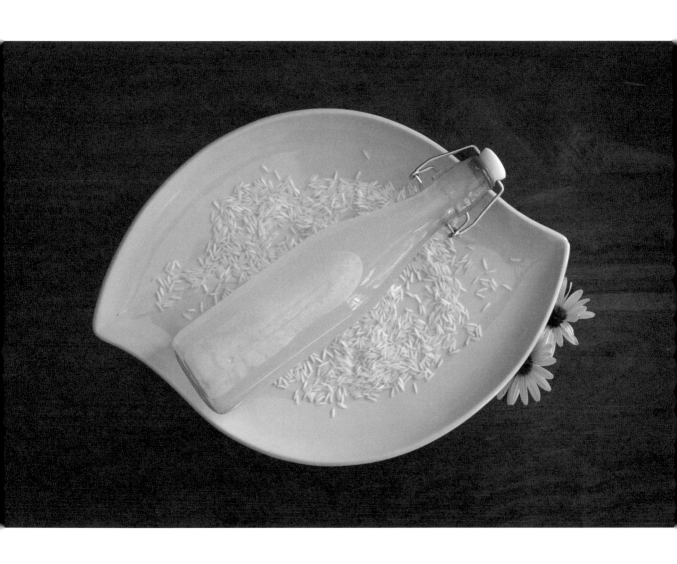

Hydrating Rice Water Hair Rinse

Shelf Life: This hair rinse will last for 7 days in the fridge.

When you cook rice, especially white rice, what do you do with the leftover water? Throw it away? Why waste that water when you can make it into a potent beauty treatment? Rice water contains antioxidants, minerals, and vitamins that will leave your hair feeling refreshed. Rice water is an excellent natural remedy for hair loss and great tool to restore hair shine. It contains inositol, which can penetrate damaged hair and repair it from the inside out. It even protects hair from future damage. Aloe vera gel is rich in vitamins A, B12, C, and E, amino acids, and fatty acids. These properties strengthen the hair and remove extra oil on the scalp. Aloe vera protects the hair from itchiness, dandruff, and adverse effects of the sun. Honey has antioxidant and humectant properties. These properties make it the perfect moisturizer for your hair. Honey ensures that your hair is soft and smooth. It also promotes hair growth and prevents hair breakage.

Ingredients

Phase	Amount	Role of Ingredient	Ingredients
Phase A	90% (90 ounces)	Foundational/functional	Leftover water from cooking rice
Phase A	5% (5 ounces)	Functional	Aloe vera gel
Phase A	5% (5 ounces)	Functional	Honey

Method

Add all ingredients to a small bottle and shake well. Apply this rinse after you wash your hair. I generally apply hair rinse after I use my conditioner.

Black Tea Hair Rinse

Shelf Life: This rinse will last for 7 days in the fridge.

Black tea has an antifungal and antibacterial effect on the hair. It protects against split ends, dryness, and brittleness by restoring moisture to the hair, which can help prevent breakage. Rose water prevents excess oil on the scalp that causes irritation and dandruff. It also serves as a moisturizer for the hair by ensuring that the scalp is moisturized. In addition, it protects the hair from heat and pollution. The vitamin A, B3, and E content of rose water soothes the scalp from irritation and itchiness because it has anti-inflammatory and antioxidant properties. Lemon peel glycerite is a potent hair-care product. It makes the hair smooth and soft while ensuring you have a clean scalp.

Ingredients

Phase	Amount	Role of Ingredient	Ingredients
Phase A	90% (90 ounces)	Foundational/functional	Black tea
Phase A	5% (5 ounces)	Functional	Lemon Peel Glycerite (page 44)
Phase A	5% (5 ounces)	Functional	Rose water or any hydrosol

Method

Add all ingredients to a small bottle and shake well. Apply this rinse after you wash your hair. I generally apply hair rinse after I use my conditioner.

Onion Peel Hair Rinse

Shelf Life: This rinse will last for 7 days in the fridge.

Onion peels contain sulfur, zinc, and calcium, which can help reduce hair loss, moisturize the scalp, and stimulate hair growth.

Ingredients

Phase	Amount	Role of Ingredient	Ingredients
Phase A	80% (80 ounces)	Foundational/functional	Leftover rice water
Phase A	10% (10 ounces)	Functional	Onion peels
Phase A	5% (5 ounces)	Functional	Aloe vera gel
Phase A	5% (5 ounces)	Functional	Apple cider vinegar

Method

Boil leftover rice water with onion peels. Once boiled, remove the peels and add the water to a spray bottle. Then, add in the remaining ingredients. Apply this product after you wash your hair. I generally apply hair rinse right after I use my conditioner.

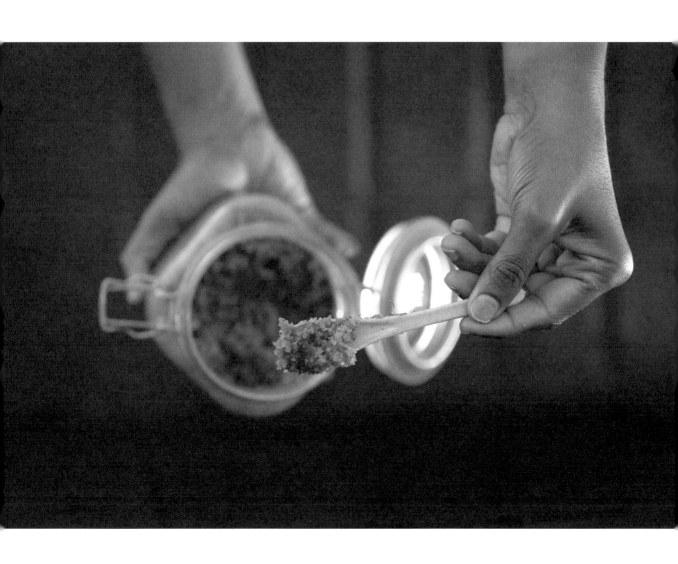

Appendix

Routines are important for beauty and wellness because they help us properly care for ourselves. Routines are especially important for those who have busy lifestyles. If you do not have time for a proper skin-care routine, you can try incorporating simple steps into your daily routine. For example, you can wash your face every morning and evening and use a moisturizer that is suitable for your skin type. You can also try using a face mask or a serum once or twice a week to boost your skin's hydration and nutrition.

If you struggle with keeping up with a beauty routine, I recommend finding a friend or family member (or app!) to help you stay on track. A beauty buddy will hold you accountable and motivate you to stick to your routine and reach your beauty goals. Healthy skin benefits your mind, body, and spirit and can spur you into making healthier choices such as drinking more water, getting more sleep, or eating better.

Without further ado, I have come up with a simple DIY sustainable beauty routine!

For Face

Step 1: Cleansing

Why we need to cleanse: Our faces are exposed to dirt, pollution, and other environmental aggressors daily. And while we may not control everything that our face comes into contact with, we can control how we cleanse it. There are many ways to cleanse your face, but sustainable beauty enthusiasts will tell you that the best way is with natural ingredients. Cleansers made with green tea, apple cider vinegar, or aloe vera juice can help cleanse your face without stripping away its natural oils. And since these ingredients are all-natural, they're gentle enough for even the most sensitive skin types. So, if you're looking for a way to step up your skin-care game, face cleansing is a great place to start.

Steps for cleansing: A single soap-based cleanse is sufficient in the morning, but I recommend double cleansing your face at night. I know it sounds counterintuitive but trust me on this one. You will take off all your makeup and/or dirt from the day with the first cleanse, then use the second cleanse to actually clean your face. It's that easy! Make sure to use a different towel for each step. Use the recipes in Chapter 5 (page 48) to develop your cleansing routine.

AM routine: Soap-based cleanser
PM routine: Oil-based cleanser followed by soap-based cleanser

Step 2: Face Toner or Facial Mist

Why we need face toner or facial mist: For anyone who's ever been skeptical about using face toner, allow me to (hopefully) convince you to give it a try. First, toner helps balance the pH of your skin after cleansing. This is important because some cleansers can actually strip away too much oil from your skin, leading to dryness, redness, and irritation. By using a toner, you can help restore the natural balance of your skin. Additionally, toners are typically very refreshing and hydrating, thanks to their water-based formulas. And if that's not enough to convince you, consider this: Regular use of face toner can also help minimize the appearance of pores and prep your skin for moisturizer and makeup. What's not to love?

Steps for toner: To make the most out of your skincare routine, use a toner after using any cleanser or soap. This will keep pores clear and hydrated for longer, helping with product absorption when applied properly and keeping impurities at bay!

AM/PM routine: Apply toner after cleansing.

Step 3: Facial Moisturizer/Serum/Oil

Why we need moisturization: If you've ever had dry skin, you know how uncomfortable it can be. Your skin may feel tight, itchy, and even flaky. An imbalance in your skin's moisture levels can lead to redness, acne, and even shiny skin from overactive oil production. So, what's the importance of moisturization? Proper hydration is key to keeping your skin looking and feeling its best. Moisturizers help lock in moisture and protect your skin from the elements. This is especially important in the colder months when the air is drier and can sap your skin of its natural moisture. There are different types of moisturizers for different skin types. If you have dry skin, you'll want to go with an oil-based cream to help hydrate and balance your skin. For those with naturally oily skin, lotions are typically a better choice since they add no extra oil to your skin. No matter what type of moisturizer you choose, make sure you're using one regularly! In short, moisturized skin is happy skin.

Steps to apply facial serum/oil: You're not alone if you've ever wondered how to apply facial serums and oils. It's a common question, and there's no one-size-fits-all answer. The best way to figure out how to apply these products is to experiment and find what works best for you. With that said, a few general tips can help guide you. First, when applying facial serum, use a pea-sized amount. Too much can lead to breakouts, as serum contains active and potent ingredients. Next, apply the serum to your face using gentle, circular motions. Once the serum is absorbed, follow up with a facial oil. Again, use a small amount and massage it into your skin using upward strokes. These products are packed with nutrients and antioxidants that your skin needs to stay healthy and looking its best, so don't be afraid to experiment until you find the application method that works best for you.

AM/PM routine: Moisturize twice a day with a facial moisturizer, serum, or oil.

Step 4: Treat Your Skin with Masks/ Peels on a Weekly Basis

Why we need weekly treatments: One of the most important things you can do for your skin is to exfoliate or apply a face mask weekly. There are plenty of good reasons to exfoliate or apply a face mask weekly. Exfoliating helps to remove dead skin cells. This can help improve your skin's overall appearance and make you look younger. Additionally, face masks can help rejuvenate your skin by providing it with essential nutrients. Applying a face mask can help improve the texture of your skin and make it look healthier. See recipes beginning on page 79.

Steps to exfoliate your face weekly: Exfoliating your face is an important part of any skin-care routine. Not only does it help remove dead

skin cells, but it also brightens the complexion and encourages cell turnover. Exfoliation can help treat a variety of skin concerns, from dullness and uneven texture to acne and premature aging. Here are a few simple steps to help you get started:

1. Start with clean, dry skin. Wet your face with warm water and apply a little cleanser to your fingertips. Gently massage your face in circular motions for about thirty seconds, then rinse with cool water. Pat your skin dry with a clean towel.

2. Apply a pea-sized amount of exfoliating scrub to your face. Add more as needed but be sure not to use too much pressure or scrub too vigorously, as this can irritate the skin. Instead, focus on using gentle, circular motions. Rinse off the scrub with cool water and pat your face dry.

3. Follow up with a hydrating serum or moisturizer. Exfoliation can strip away natural oils, so it's important to replenish the skin afterwards. Look for hyaluronic acid or glycerin-based products to help lock in moisture. Apply them while your skin is still damp for the best results.

Steps to apply a face mask weekly: Applying a face mask is a great way to give your skin a little extra TLC. Here are a few tips to get the most out of your masking session:

1. Always apply your mask to freshly cleansed skin. This will help ensure that your pores are clear and allow the mask to penetrate your skin better.
2. A little goes a long way with face masks. You only need to apply a thin layer to see results.
3. Don't forget to extend the mask down to your neck. This area is often neglected, but it also needs some love!
4. Once you've applied your face mask, take a few minutes to relax. Put on some soothing music, grab a book, and spend ten to fifteen minutes letting the mask work its magic.
5. When you're ready, rinse off the mask with lukewarm water. Avoid using hot water, as this can dry out your skin. Follow up with your favorite moisturizer.

Step 5: Protect your Skin with Sunscreen

No matter your skin type, sunscreen should always be a necessary part of your beauty routine. This is one product I strongly urge you *not* to make yourself because it's nearly impossible to get the same consistency and quality through a DIY process. Sunscreen works by absorbing or reflecting the sun's rays, and choosing a formula suited for your specific skin type is important. For example, if you have dry skin, you will want to look for a sunscreen that is noncomedogenic and contains hydrating ingredients like glycerin or hyaluronic acid. If you have oily skin, you will want to look for a lightweight formula that won't clog your pores. No matter what your skin type, there is a sunscreen out there that will work for you, so don't forget to apply it every day!

There are two main types of sunscreen: physical and chemical. Physical sunscreens work by sitting on top of the skin and reflecting UV rays away from the body. Chemical sunscreens work by absorbing UV rays and converting them into heat energy. Both types of sunscreen are effective at protecting against the harmful effects of UV exposure, but they each have their benefits and drawbacks. Physical sunscreens are generally considered more natural and gentler on the skin. They are also longer lasting, making them ideal for activities like swimming or sweating. However, they can sometimes be thick and difficult to apply evenly, leaving streaks or white patches on the skin. Chemical sunscreens are typically lighter and easier to apply evenly. They also absorb more easily into the skin, making them less likely to irritate. However, they may not be as long-lasting as physical sunscreens, and some people find them more drying.

Ultimately, it's up to each individual to decide which type of sunscreen is right for them. Both have their pros and cons, so it's important to choose the one that best fits your needs.

Basic Beauty Tips for Your Hands and Feet

Here are a few simple things you can do to keep your hands and feet looking and feeling their best.

1. Wash your hands regularly with soap and water and dry them thoroughly.
2. Apply lotion to your hands and feet after washing them while they're still damp. This will help lock in moisture.
3. Wear gloves when doing any activities that involve getting your hands wet, such as dishes or gardening.
4. Wear socks and shoes that fit well and aren't too tight. This will help prevent blisters.
5. Trim your nails regularly and file them down if they get too long. Long nails can cause problems such as ingrown nails.
6. If you have any cuts or scrapes on your hands or feet, clean them well and bandage them up to prevent infection.

Basic Beauty Tips for Your Nails

Your nails comprise layers of a protein called keratin. As new cells grow at the base of your nails, older cells harden and flatten out, forming the visible part of your nail. To prevent problems, taking good care of your nails and cuticles is important. Here are some tips:

1. Wash your hands with soap and water regularly. This will help remove dirt and bacteria from under your nails.
2. Use a mild shampoo when you wash your hair to avoid drying out your nails and cuticles.
3. Trim your nails regularly and file them down if they get too long. Longer nails are more likely to get broken or chipped.
4. Be gentle when cleaning under your nails. Don't dig too deep and damage the tissue around your nails.
5. Moisturize your hands and feet often, especially if they are dry. This will help keep your nails and cuticles healthy.
6. Wear gloves when doing chores involving water or harsh chemicals. This will protect your nails from drying out or getting damaged.
7. See your doctor if you have any concerns about your nails such as changes in color or texture or pain

around your nails. These could be signs of a more serious problem.

Daily Face Routine

Step 1: Facial cleanser (either soap, gel, or foam)
Step 2: Facial toner (to balance the pH of the skin)
Step 3: Facial moisturizer, serum, or oil
Step 4: Treat your skin weekly by exfoliating or applying a facial mask
Step 5: Protect, protect, protect with sunscreen

Nightly Face Routine

Step 1: Double facial cleanser (use a bi-phase or oil-based cleanser first, then follow with a gel- or foam-based cleanser)
Step 2: Facial toner (to balance the pH of the skin)
Step 3: Facial serum, oil, or moisturizer

Sustainable Hair-care Steps to Consider

Maintaining healthy hair is more than just washing and conditioning it regularly. Your diet, stress levels, medication, or supplements can all affect how your locks look! Here are a few pointers for an ideal hair-care routine:

Step 1: Hair cleansing (shampoo), ideally twice a week
Step 2: Hair conditioning, ideally twice a week
Step 3: Hair oiling, preferred weekly
Step 4: Hair moisturizing (leave-in conditioners), based on hair type
Step 5: Styling products; I prefer natural products, as store-brought styling products can be toxic
Step 5: Hair care (hair mask, hair rinse, etc.), based on your hair type

Sustainable Body-care Steps to Consider

An ideal body-care routine should encompass all aspects of self-care, from taking care of your skin to exercising and eating healthy. While there is no one-size-fits-all approach to body care, everyone should follow a few basic principles. First, cleanse your skin regularly. This will remove dirt, oil, and impurities that can clog pores and lead to breakouts. Second, exfoliate your skin regularly. This will help slough away dead skin cells and reveal brighter, more radiant skin. Third, moisturize your skin daily. This will help prevent dryness and keep your skin looking supple and youthful. Finally, don't forget to protect your skin from the sun with sunscreen. By following these simple steps, you can maintain healthy, beautiful skin for years.

We all have those days where we feel like we can't get out of bed, let alone face the world. When we're feeling low, it's important to remember that taking care of our bodies is as important as taking care of our minds. A simple body-care routine can make all the difference. Here are a few things you can do to show your body some love:

- Take a relaxing bath
- Moisturize your skin
- Give yourself a foot massage
- Eat healthy foods
- Drink plenty of water
- Get enough sleep

By pampering your body, you'll be surprised at how much better you'll feel overall. So. add body care to your self-care routine—you deserve it! Here is my suggested body-care routine:

Step 1: Dry brushing (massaging the skin with a dry, stiff-bristled brush without any oil or lotion), ideally twice a week. The skin is typically brushed toward the heart, starting at the hands and feet, and brushing toward the chest. It is generally performed before you take a shower. This at-home treatment is considered detoxifying, circulation-stimulating, and body-toning.

Step 2: Prewash body massage (abhyanga), ideally twice a week

Step 3: Body cleansing, daily (typically in the bath or shower)

Step 4: Body exfoliating (using a body scrub), once a week

Step 5: Body moisturizers, daily (ideally after a bath or shower)

Step 6: Body masks or any other body therapies, once a month

Step 7: Nail care, ideally once a week, but if you are moisturizing nails regularly, every other week works just as well

Beauty Inside Out: Clean Eating for Clear Skin and Gut Health

You are what you eat, so they say. And never is that truer than when it comes to your skin and gut health. The food you put into your body has a direct impact on the way your skin looks and feels. If you want to have clear, glowing skin, you need to start from the inside out by eating clean.

Clean eating is all about consuming whole, unprocessed foods. That means lots of fruits, vegetables, lean proteins, and healthy fats. Processed foods are full of sugar, artificial ingredients, and unhealthy fats that can wreak havoc on your skin. They can cause inflammation, breakouts, and dull, lifeless skin. Clean eating supports gut health, which is essential for clear skin. A healthy gut means happy skin! When your gut is full of unhealthy bacteria, it can lead to inflammation, breakouts, and dull skin. But when your gut is healthy and balanced, your skin will reflect that. Here are some tips for eating clean:

1. Fill up on fruits and vegetables. Fruits and vegetables are packed with vitamins, minerals, and antioxidants that are essential for clear skin. Aim to eat at least five servings of fruits and vegetables per day. That may seem like a lot, but it's actually not that difficult. A serving of fruit is about 1 cup, whereas a serving of vegetables is about ½ cup. An easy way to get your five servings is to have a large salad for lunch and a piece of fruit with breakfast and snacks.

2. Choose lean proteins. Lean proteins are an important part of a clean diet. They help build and repair skin tissue, and they also contain amino acids that support gut health. Good sources of lean protein include chicken, fish, tofu, legumes, and eggs.

3. Limit processed foods and sugar. Processed foods and sugar can cause inflammation, breakouts, and dull skin. So, it's best to limit them as much as possible. This doesn't mean you have to completely eliminate them from your diet but try to eat them in moderation.

4. Drink plenty of water. Water is essential for clear skin. It helps to flush out toxins and keep your skin hydrated. Aim to drink eight glasses of water per day.

5. Eat probiotic-rich foods. Probiotics are good bacteria that support gut health. They can be found in fermented foods like yogurt, kimchi, and sauerkraut. You can also take a probiotic supplement if you don't like fermented foods.

Clean eating is a simple yet effective way to get clear skin. By filling up on whole, unprocessed foods, you'll be supporting gut health and giving your skin the nutrients it needs to thrive. So, ditch the processed foods and sugar, and start eating clean for clear skin!

Frequently Asked Questions (FAQs)

Where do I get all these ingredients from?
Even though we use food peels and seeds a lot, there are a few ingredients you might need to buy and stock as needed. At the time of my writing, I found most ingredients from Amazon or natural supermarkets.

If I only want to make 2 ounces of wintery cuticle oil from this book, how do I do it?
To make 2 ounces of wintery cuticle oil, see the section on calculating DIY recipes on page 10.

I want to make a recipe but don't have one ingredient. Is there any replacement for something similar?
Absolutely! I encourage you to be courageous while stirring up your beauty products. Please research essential oil before replacing them or increasing the amount.

What's the difference between natural and organic, especially in terms of beauty products?
All organic ingredients are natural, but not all natural ingredients are organic. To identify truly organic beauty products, look for the USDA NOP-certified organic seal or ECOCERT label.

The beauty industry uses the term "natural" loosely. To my knowledge, there is no regulated stamp or seal for natural beauty products. When a brand says that their products are all natural, that does not necessarily mean they are not using synthetic ingredients like emulsifiers, surfactants, and preservatives. They may use these artificial ingredients along with some natural ingredients.

What's the difference between recipes on the Internet versus the ones in this book?
There is a lot of good content on the Internet, but many online beauty recipes are written by amateurs who unknowingly share unsafe practices. I adopt a beauty chemist's approach to the recipes in this book. If you follow my principles of sustainable beauty, you can be sure that whatever you make will remain safe and effective for your skin.

Since I have used no preservatives, what should I do with a large batch of face toner?

It's always good to refrigerate water-based beauty products. If you refrigerate it, use it within a week or freeze it. Regarding preservatives, I want to share that, as human beings, we are being told that no-preservative foods are better for us, but with skin-care products, it's not good to use unpreserved skin care. Storing it in the refrigerator stops microbial/bacterial processes, which can eventually damage the skin-care products if left unchecked.

Will my DIY products be as effective as store-bought products?

Yes, my DIY recipes are well-measured and provide you with total control over what goes into your product. You get rid of fillers like water by giving your skin a DIY dose.

What's the shelf life of oils and butters?

If you're anything like me, you have a cupboard full of different oils and butters, each with a slightly different expiration date. It can be a little overwhelming trying to keep track of them all because all oils and butters have different shelf lives. It can vary from three months to five years so, to be safe, check the specific oil or butter's expiration date before use.

It's too much information. How do I start my DIY skin-care journey?

Start with slow steps if you feel overwhelmed with the DIY skin-care journey. Slow change is more sustainable than radical change. I recommend choosing which product(s) you can most easily develop and incorporate into your beauty regimen.

Can I make sunscreen at home?

The short answer is no! It's not possible to DIY, as we can't run any lab tests on DIY products. The ingredients in sunscreen create a physical barrier on your skin that reflects UV rays away from your body. Look for a sunscreen with at least SPF 30 and reapply it every two hours or more often if you're sweating or swimming. Sunscreen containing zinc oxide will give you a white film on your skin. If you are not fan of that, consider chemical sunscreen.

What is sustainable beauty?

The definition you will see everywhere on the Internet is that sustainability is the long-term ability to meet needs without destroying resources or damaging ecosystem functions such as clean water supply, agriculture production, and protection from pollution. I define sustainability or sustainable beauty as simply living within your means and achieving this through intelligent consumption habits that promote thriftiness while

simultaneously looking out for yourself, both
financially, emotionally, mentally, etc.

**Where can we find your other recipes and
beauty and wellness wisdom?**
You can find me at glowngreen.com.
My Instagram handle is @glowngreen
You can reach out to me personally via
contact@glowngreen.com.

About the Author

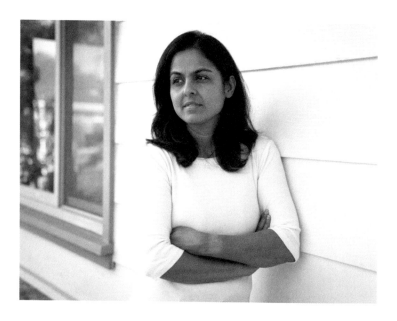

Ruchita Acharya is a beauty blogger, a small business owner, and the creative mind behind *Glow & Green*. Ruchita's mission is to empower women with the tools to transition to a sustainable lifestyle, explicitly focusing on beauty and personal care. Through her platform, Ruchita shares recipes to teach people how to make their products at home: from soaps and shampoo bars to customizable facial potions. Ruchita also opened an online store from which she sells her soaps, facial oils, bath scrubs, and other sustainable skincare products made from food by-products. She also hosts beauty workshops in the San Francisco Bay Area where she demos how to make all-natural beauty products. Attendees get to take home samples of what they made in class. In addition to beauty blogging and running her small business, Ruchita moonlights as a freelance writer and consultant on sustainable beauty.

Index

lip scrub
    Grapefruit Peel Lip Scrub, 82

M
Mango Seed Face Mask, 79
mango seed powder
    Mango Seed Face Mask, 79
manufacturing practices, 27–34
mask
    body
        Mojito Body Mask, 122
    face, 177–178
        Brightening Face Mask, 89
    hair and scalp, 144–155
matcha powder
    Emulsified Pistachio Matcha Scrub,
        114
microbeads, 5
microplastics, 5
middle notes, 19
Mint Choco Foot Balm, 127
mint stem-infused almond oil
    Mint Choco Foot Balm, 127
mint stem-infused apricot kernel oil
    Sesame Hair Oil, 165
mint stem-infused grapeseed oil
    Anhydrous Minty Moisturizer, 61
    Salty Herbal Scrub, 115–116
mint stem-infused sunflower oil
    Herby Facial Oil, 65
    Minty Choco Body Butter for Dry
        Skin, 107
Minty Choco Body Butter for Dry
    Skin, 107
mist, facial, 176
moisturizers
    body, 102–112
    facial, 60–66, 176–177
Mojito Body Mask, 122
Moringa Herby Soap Base, 99–100
Multani mitti, 24
My Go-To Leave-In Conditioner, 139
My Go-To Walnutty Soapy Scrub, 119

N
nail care, 179–180
notes, of essential oils, 19–20
Nutty Hair Scrub, 152

O
oatmeal
    Dry Ayurvedic Soap Powder, 93
oil(s)
    apricot kernel, 14
    argan, 15
        Wrinkle-Free Oil Serum, 63
    aromas of, 19–20
    avocado, 14
    carrier, 12–16, 20
    castor, 14
        Fruity Facial Oil, 66
        Hydrating Oil for Hair Growth,
            166
    chemistry of, 13
    coconut, 14
        Emulsified Pistachio Matcha
            Scrub, 114
        Fruity Facial Oil, 66
        Grapefruit Peel Lip Scrub, 82
        Hydrating Oil for Hair Growth,
            166
        Mojito Body Mask, 122
        Turmeric Body Mask (Ubtan),
            121
    cold-pressed, 13
    combining water and, 29
    essential, 18–22
    facial, 60–66
    grapeseed, 15
        Anhydrous Minty Moisturizer, 61
        Creamy Liquid Soap, 97
    heated extraction of, 13
    infusions with, 41–42
    jojoba, 15
    neem, 15
    olive, 14
    pomegranate, 15–16
    rosehip, 15
        Carrot Peel Facial Cleanser, 59
    sunflower, 14–15
        Herby Facial Oil, 65
    sweet almond, 14
    unrefined, 13
Oil-Free Facial Lotion Spray, 64
Onion Peel Hair Rinse, 173
onion peel-infused coconut oil
    Sesame Hair Oil, 165

onion peels
    Henna Hair Dye, 159–161
    Onion Peel Hair Rinse, 173
orange essential oil, 20
    Fruity Facial Oil, 66
    Orange Peel Cleansing Balm, 57–58
    Orange Peel Foot Soak, 129
    Probiotic Citrusy Gel Soap, 94
Orange Peel Cleansing Balm, 57–58
Orange Peel Foot Soak, 129
orange peel glycerite
    Dark Circle-Removng Eye Gel, 69
orange peel-infused almond oil
    Fruity Hair Balm, 167
    Hydrating Oil for Hair Growth, 166
    Orange Peel Cleansing Balm, 57–58
orange peel powder
    Dry Rub Almond-Turmeric Scrub,
        115–116
    Orange Peel Foot Soak, 129
    Powdered Ayurvedic Hair Mask,
        149
    Turmeric Body Mask (Ubtan), 121
orange peels
    Fruit Scraps Facial Steam, 74
orange peel tincture, 46
oriental aromas, 19
Overnight Hair Mask, 151

P
palm oil, 5
parabens, 4–5
parsley stem-infused sunflower oil
    Herby Facial Oil, 65
parsley stem powder
    Green Shampoo Bars, 137
    Moringa Herby Soap Base, 99–100
patch test, 26
pineapple peel powder
    Mojito Body Mask, 122
pistachio shell powder, 45
    Emulsified Pistachio Matcha Scrub,
        114
    Foamy Exfoliating Cleanser, 55
    Nutty Hair Scrub, 152
plastics, 5
plastic wrap, 30
pollution, 5